ENJOY YOUR LABOR

A New Approach to Pain Relief for Childbirth

ENJOY YOUR LABOR

A New Approach to Pain Relief for Childbirth

Gilbert J. Grant, MD

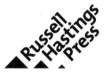

White Plains, New York
www.russellhastingspress.com

Enjoy Your Labor: A New Approach to Pain Relief for Childbirth.

Published by Russell Hastings Press, Ltd.

P.O. Box 229, White Plains, New York 10605

Russell Hastings Press books may be purchased for educational, business, or promotional use. For information, contact Russell Hastings Press, Ltd. in writing at P.O. Box 229, White Plains, NY 10605 or by e mail at sales@RussellHastingsPress.com.

Library of Congress Cataloging-in-Publication Data

Grant, Gilbert J., 1956–

Enjoy Your Labor: A New Approach to Pain Relief for Childbirth

First edition, Second printing

p.   cm.

Includes Glossary and Index

ISBN 0-9759939-0-9

Library of Congress Control Number: 2004097972

1. Childbirth   2. Pregnancy   3. Anesthesia

Cartoon Illustrations by David Zinn

Medical Illustrations by P. Jasmine Katatikarn

Visit www.EnjoyYourLabor.com for
educational video animations and additional information.

BEFORE YOU BEGIN READING...

CONTENTS

ACKNOWLEDGMENTS

The publication of *Enjoy Your Labor* would not have been possible were it not for the help of many people. Acknowledging specific individuals for their contributions is inherently risky, because others may be inadvertently omitted. But with this caveat in mind, here goes.

It is difficult to imagine completing this book without the sage advice, guidance and hard work of my father and my teacher, Abraham H. Grant, MD. His tireless assistance, encouragement, contributions and input at every stage of the writing and production of *Enjoy Your Labor* cannot be overstated. But more important than the enormous effort he expended on the book itself has been his role in molding my character. By his instruction, and even more so by his example, my father's genuine concern for his patients has indelibly shaped my approach to relieving the suffering of women in labor.

There are many others who provided support, suggestions, and encouragement throughout the long process of writing this book. I would be remiss if I did not mention my dear friends Shivi Isman, Jessica R. Friedman and Amy Erani, multitalented women who provided invaluable assistance with this project. Many relatives selflessly contributed their time and talents including my brother-in-law Alan Granader and my aunt Libby Newman. Numerous professional friends and colleagues were also instrumental in offering advice, criticism and suggestions. Without doubt, their collective input and critiques strengthened the finished product. In particular, Dr. Jerome Lax, a close friend and colleague in anesthesiology, provided considerable insightful counsel.

My philosophy of providing pain relief for women giving birth, and my dedication to caring for them was in no small part influenced by a wonderful human being and a great clinician, Dr. Sivam Ramanathan, my mentor in obstetric anesthesia. And as I wrote this book my thoughts often drifted to a spectacular obstetrician-gynecologist who influenced my career choice and delivered my daughters: Dr. Ken Weissman, my late brother-in-law.

Last, but by no means least, this book would not have been possible without the consistent support and understanding of my wife Judy and my three daughters: Alexandra, Tori, and Sydney. With understanding and without complaining (much), they tolerated my absence from their midst as I worked on *Enjoy Your Labor*. Their support was crucial in seeing the project through.

New York, N.Y.
December 2004

PREFACE

Why I Wrote This Book
and
Why You Should Read It

As an anesthesiologist, I have been caring for women during labor and delivery for 20 years. I specialize in relieving the pain of childbirth using the most effective and reliable means available—epidurals and spinals. In my experience, I've noticed that many mothers-to-be are concerned about the safety of these pain relief techniques. The thought of receiving an epidural, which involves inserting a needle into the lower back, can be very unsettling. The mere mention of the term "spinal" may cause even more fear, often compounded by having heard a frightening story about anesthesia. A woman's double-edged fear, of both labor pain and the techniques commonly used to treat it, can cause anxiety for months before delivery.

Women attending childbirth education classes, who are predominantly first-time mothers-to-be, report that some instructors put a negative spin on epidurals and spinals, dismissing them as "unnatural" or even harmful interventions. Social pressures may needlessly dissuade women from choosing an epidural or spinal if they feel that a request for pain relief will be interpreted as a sign of weakness. Women also refrain from asking for pain medication out of concern that it will harm their babies—an unnecessary fear, mixed with guilt.

Beyond these issues, I came to realize that the leading cause of misunderstandings about modern pain relief techniques is simply a lack of accurate and up-to-date information. Browsing through the books my wife read during her first pregnancy,

1

I found that although many of them discussed a variety of ways to manage the pain of childbirth, none presented the full picture of epidurals and spinals, even though these methods are used by most women who give birth in the United States. Worse still, I found that some books were filled with erroneous information about these techniques.

In 1996, to better inform and educate patients about epidurals and spinals, I began offering a monthly seminar at New York University Medical Center, where I work and teach. The success of this program persuaded me to extend its reach by writing this book. *Enjoy Your Labor* is based on the questions that expectant mothers have asked me over the years. It describes epidural and spinal techniques in detail. It demystifies these procedures by explaining in easy-to-understand terms exactly what to expect. Once women have a thorough understanding of what's involved, I have found that they are much less anxious about receiving pain relief, and perhaps about the process of delivery itself.

In addition to presenting incomplete and inaccurate information about epidurals and spinals, however, there is something else missing from other books: not one describes the "new" approach to labor pain relief that I recommend. My philosophy is quite simple. It is based on common sense: if you choose to have the best pain relief possible for labor and delivery (an epidural and/or a spinal), you should receive it *before* severe pain begins, assuming it has been established that you are in labor. Unfortunately, most women today receive the epidural *after* their labor pain becomes unbearable. Although my approach seems obvious and logical, many people oppose it, perhaps because it is so radically different from the way childbirth pain has been handled for so long. After reading this book, you'll understand why it makes sense to get the epidural as soon as it is clear that you are truly in labor, and before the pain becomes intolerable.

I chose the title *Enjoy Your Labor* because that is what I tell my patients after I give them their epidural. You *can* enjoy your labor, by educating yourself about the types of pain relief you may choose, and by taking advantage of what modern medicine has to offer. After reading this book — well in advance of your due date — talk to your obstetrician or midwife about your concerns regarding labor pain relief and the available options. If you require additional information, contact an anesthesiologist at the hospital where you are planning to deliver your baby. To help you feel at ease about your upcoming childbirth, it makes sense to discuss the alternatives with the people who will be assisting you through labor and delivery.

This book is written from my perspective as an obstetric anesthesiologist practicing in a major teaching hospital where medical advances are introduced, and where my colleagues and I provide full-time coverage in the labor and delivery suite. At smaller facilities, anesthesiologists may serve obstetric patients on an as-needed basis: certain techniques described in this book may not be available at such places. Learn which options will be available to you by speaking with both your obstetric care provider and an anesthesiologist where you will be delivering long before labor commences.

A clear understanding of the process of labor pain relief will reduce your fears about your upcoming delivery. Empower yourself with knowledge so that you can make an informed choice. Furthermore, knowing what to expect in terms of pain management will help to focus your thoughts on the one that is most important: the anticipation of your new baby.

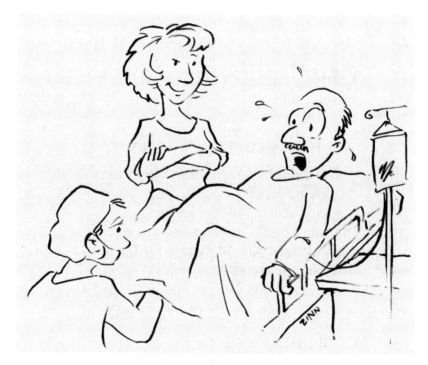

A sure way for women to experience painless childbirth

1

PERCEPTIONS OF CHILDBIRTH PAIN RELIEF

Topics Due to be Delivered

- Is a double standard in effect for women giving birth?
- Is "natural" always better?
- The role of guilt in childbirth pain relief
- Every woman should decide for herself whether she wants pain relief

THE DOUBLE STANDARD

Imagine this: you are being wheeled in to have your appendix removed when a member of the surgical team peers down from above his mask and says, "Tell you what we'll do. Bear up as best you can without anesthesia, and if it gets too rough we'll give you something for the pain." Sounds crazy, right? No man would be asked to submit to an appendectomy, which can be performed in 24 minutes, without anesthesia. Yet the severe pain of labor, which can persist for more than 24 hours, is somehow viewed as a condition that women should simply endure, since childbirth is a natural process — as if "natural" pain is any less intense than that induced by a surgeon's scalpel. In fact, the pain of childbirth is the worst pain that most women will experience in their entire lives.

So why is there so much prejudice against epidurals and spinals? Part of the explanation is that women are often treated as second-class citizens. How else can one explain why pain relief for labor is still considered an option or a luxury? Menstrual cramps, which pale in comparison to labor contractions, are routinely treated with pain relievers. So why does anyone question whether labor pain merits treatment? As more than a few women have observed, if men had labor pain, its relief would probably be viewed quite differently.

The Huichol Indians of north-central Mexico sought to make childbirth a more equitable experience. Their interesting birthing practice, illustrated in Figure 1-1, intimately involved the father-to-be in the process. "According to Huichol tradition, when a woman had her first child, the husband squatted in the rafters of the house, or in the branches of a tree, directly above her, with ropes attached to his scrotum. As she went into labor pain, the wife pulled vigorously on the ropes, so that her husband shared in the painful, but ultimately joyous, experience of childbirth."[1]

NATURAL OR UNNATURAL?

The term "natural" implies that a birth in which the mother receives pain medication is somehow "unnatural." Who would ever choose an "unnatural" childbirth? However, the term "unnatural" sounds plain silly when applied to, for example, pneumonia, for which you could choose the "unnatural" approach and take penicillin, or do it the "natural" way and die. Granted, these two situations are not identical: unlike untreated pneumonia, the pain of labor and delivery will not kill anyone. However, I attach no less importance to the suffering of a woman in labor than to the suffering of a patient with pneumonia: both situations deserve treatment if the individual who is suffering desires it.

I vividly recall a conversation with a physician who told me that, in his practice, laboring women are informed that the pain

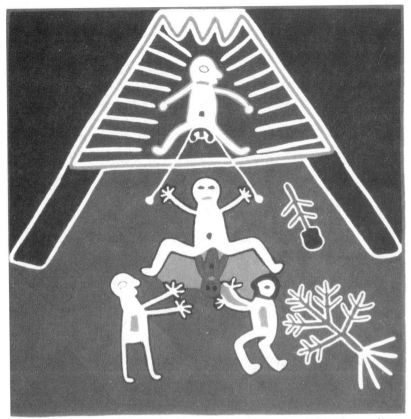

Fig. 1-1. *How the husband assists in the birth of a child. The tradition of the Huichol Indians of north-central Mexico. Reproduced with permission of the Fine Arts Museums of San Francisco.*

they are experiencing is a natural part of childbirth, and that once they understand this, the pain is much more bearable. Interesting, I thought. If someone told me the severe pain I was experiencing was natural, I do not think it would hurt any less: I would want relief, and quickly!

Pregnant Pause

"Natural" pain may hurt just as much or even more than "unnatural" pain. Both can be treated—if that's what you want.

Natural childbirth preparation may be a set-up for feeling inadequate. This is because some childbirth educators teach that if you learn the breathing and focusing techniques and practice them properly, you'll be able to avoid pain medication. For many mothers-to-be, this approach is doomed to fail because in reality, breathing and focusing cannot eliminate the pain. So when the woman in labor breathes and focuses but still experiences pain, she may think that it is all her fault: "If only I had paid more attention in class and learned how to do the breathing better, it wouldn't hurt now." If she ends up asking for and receiving an epidural, she may feel even more of a failure.

Epidural Episodes:
BIRTH PANGS AND PANGS OF CONSCIENCE

F.S. was a first-time mother-to-be who was convinced that she did not want any type of pain medication for labor. She was highly motivated, and had dutifully attended a childbirth education course. Her labor pains gradually became more intense and ultimately much more severe than she had imagined they would be. She did her breathing and focusing that she had learned, but found that the intensity of her labor pain was no match for the techniques she was using to cope with them. But she was determined to avoid an epidural. It was only after six agonizing hours that she finally tired of her pain, and pleaded for an epidural. We immediately gave her one, which worked as it was intended to, relieving all of her pain within 15 minutes. I thought that she would be pleased, now that we had ended her agony, but I was mistaken. When I visited her room half-an-hour later she was crying uncontrollably — out of guilt for having taken the epidural. What a scene: she was completely comfortable, no longer feeling her contractions but she thought she had failed her "test." This dramatically demonstrates the problem with "natural" approaches: a woman is made to feel a failure if she asks for pain relief.

FEELINGS OF GUILT

Mothers-to-be are often made to feel guilty for asking for pain relief. This attitude is inappropriate, especially in light of the recent advances that have been made in obstetric anesthesia, and improvements in epidural and spinal techniques. Nevertheless, this thinking persists in our culture, along with numerous myths and misconceptions about modern techniques for relieving childbirth pain. One example of this is the belief that modern anesthesia is an "easy way out" that compromises the safety of both mother and child. As you will see after reading this book, not only are epidurals and spinals safe for the overwhelming majority of mothers and their babies, mothers who do not use them may be exposing themselves to unnecessary risks. These risks, which usually are not even considered, are discussed in Chapter Eight.

Pregnant Pause

Consider your options for pain relief carefully before labor begins. When you are in the throes of labor pain, you will not be in the best condition to weigh these options objectively.

ONLY YOU CAN JUDGE

Pain is a completely subjective sensation, so no one else can judge how much or how little you are experiencing. Individuals not in labor (doctors, midwives, nurses and coaches) tend to underestimate the intensity of the woman's pain and suffering; yet these are the people who often advise her whether she should take something for the pain. This process begins long before labor: childbirth educators often mislead women about the severity of the pain that they will experience during labor and delivery. In discussing how some individuals downplay the severity of the pain, Dr. Peter Brownridge, an Australian anesthesiologist, wrote: "To pretend, therefore, that natural childbirth is other than very painful for most women can only be described as a cruel and callous deception."[2] Learn about what to expect during labor and delivery, and find out what options are available, so that you can make an informed decision about what type of pain relief, if any, you want.

Key Concepts to Carry Away

Although many women are made to feel guilty for wanting to relieve the pain of childbirth, most end up requesting and receiving epidurals and/or spinals. Don't let anyone else make the decision for you. Empower yourself by obtaining the knowledge that you need to decide what type of pain relief, if any, will be best for you when you deliver your baby.

2

CAUSES OF CHILDBIRTH PAIN AND STRATEGIES FOR ITS RELIEF

Topics Due to be Delivered

- **The origins of pain during the different stages of labor and delivery**
- **Two different approaches to pain relief: systemic versus regional**
- **Why regional pain relief is the most effective option for childbirth**

THE BASIS FOR PAIN

What is the cause of pain? Why does something hurt? Pain begins when a part of the body is cut, stretched, pressed, or exposed to heat or extreme cold. This starts a pain message that travels through the nerves—the body's communication system—first to the spinal cord and then up to the brain. When the message arrives in the brain we perceive the pain. This entire process happens in less than a second.

THE STAGES OF LABOR AND PERCEPTION OF PAIN

The pain message originates from different locations as labor progresses. Labor is divided into three stages. It begins with the onset of regular uterine contractions, which cause the cervix, the outlet at the base of the uterus through which the baby passes into the vagina, to dilate (open). The first stage of labor ends when the cervix is fully dilated to a diameter of 10 centimeters. Pain during the first stage is caused by contractions of the uterus and stretching of the cervix. At the beginning of labor, the contractions produce a sensation that is at first uncomfortable, often likened to bad menstrual cramps, but which gradually becomes more intense. Women perceive first stage pains in different locations, most commonly in the lower abdomen, but many also feel them in their back. Some also feel the pain in their buttocks, hips, and thighs.

When the cervix is dilated to about seven or eight centimeters the pain becomes even more intense. During this interval, known as "transition"—that is, the transition from the first to the second stage of labor—some women experience nausea and vomiting.

During the second stage, as the baby descends through the birth canal, pain is caused in two ways: by the contracting uterus and also by the stretching—and sometimes the tearing—of tissue in the cervix, vagina and perineum (the area between the vagina and the anus). The second stage of labor, also known as the pushing stage, ends with the delivery of the baby. The third stage is the interval between the birth of the baby and delivery of the placenta.

WHEN WILL LABOR PAIN START AND HOW SEVERE WILL IT BE?

Each woman has a unique experience with labor pain. Some women have more pain earlier in labor; a very few never experience much pain at all. In general, the pain of early contractions is less severe than the pain that occurs later as labor progresses. The intensity and location of the pain may also depend on the baby's position as it descends through the birth canal. For example, if the baby's head is positioned to emerge face up, the mother is more likely to have pain in the lower back ("back labor").

SYSTEMIC VERSUS REGIONAL PAIN RELIEF

There are two different approaches used to treat the pain of childbirth with medication: systemic and regional. With the systemic approach, the medication is given throughout the entire "system" (body) of the mother-to-be, and a portion makes its way to the brain where it blunts the perception of pain. With the regional approach, a relatively small dose of medication is given into a specific "region" of the body (the epidural or spinal space) to block the pain message from being transmitted up to the brain.

SYSTEMIC PAIN RELIEF

The systemic drugs most commonly used in labor are the narcotics Demerol, morphine, Stadol and Nubain. They are injected into a vein or a muscle and they exert their effects in the brain to diminish perception of pain. Because little technical expertise is required to administer systemic medication, their use does not require the presence of an anesthesiologist, so if an anesthesiologist is not available, the systemic approach makes sense.

But the systemic approach has many disadvantages. Patients tend to feel drowsy after receiving systemically-administered narcotics. Nausea and vomiting often occur. Furthermore, because a relatively large dose is used, a considerable amount of the drug may be transferred to the baby, making the newborn sleepy and slowing his or her breathing.

The main downside of systemic narcotics is that they do not relieve labor pain effectively. They often cause the mother-to-be to fall asleep between contractions, only to have her wake up groaning during contractions. Once it is established that a woman is truly in labor, there is no reason to use systemic narcotics unless she is not able to receive an epidural or a spinal for a specific medical reason. These reasons are listed in Chapter Seven.

Pregnant Pause

If the pain message is stopped in its tracks before it is transmitted up to the brain, pain will not be perceived. This is how regional pain relief techniques — epidurals and spinals — work. The advantage of a regional approach is that the mother is awake, alert, pain-free and able to actively participate in the birth.

REGIONAL PAIN RELIEF

The regional approach is fundamentally different from the systemic approach. With regional pain relief, the medication is administered directly into the epidural or spinal space. In this way, the pain message is stopped before it has a chance to travel up the spinal cord, so it never reaches the brain.

With spinals and epidurals, since the medication is injected directly into the area where it is needed to relieve the pain, much smaller doses are used compared to the systemic approach, and therefore there are fewer side effects. The mother's state of mind is not altered, and the smaller doses mean that very little medication reaches the baby. The technical aspects of spinal and epidural techniques are described in detail in Chapter Three.

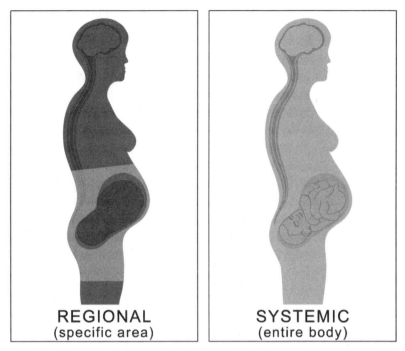

| REGIONAL | SYSTEMIC |
| (specific area) | (entire body) |

Fig. 2-1. *Regional versus systemic pain relief. The lighter shade indicates areas affected by the medication. With regional pain relief, a specific area of the body is numbed, and the baby is unaffected. With systemic pain relief, the entire body is affected, including the baby.*

Key Concepts to Carry Away

Regional pain relief techniques, epidurals and spinals, are based on the administration of small doses of anesthetics very close to the location of the nerves that carry the pain message. The result is a pain-free mother-to-be and a vigorous newborn. If labor pain is severe enough to warrant treatment, why not choose the most effective means available to get maximal pain relief with a minimum of side effects for you and your baby?

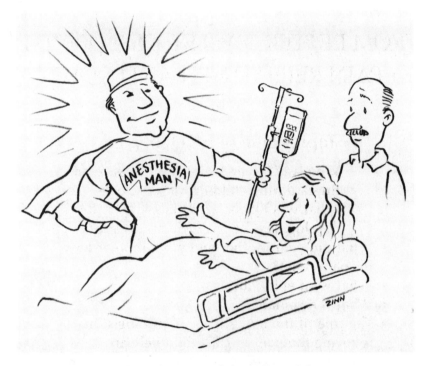

"Where have you been all my life?"

3

FROM BETTER TO BEST: CHILDBIRTH PAIN RELIEF THEN AND NOW

 ## Topics Due to be Delivered

- Who was the first American to have anesthesia during childbirth?
- What was Queen Victoria's role in the development of obstetric anesthesia?
- What did your mother and grandmother have for pain relief?
- What is an epidural?
- What is a spinal?
- The role of the modern anesthesiologist in relieving the pain of labor and delivery

HISTORY OF CHILDBIRTH PAIN RELIEF

Pain relief for childbirth followed the introduction of ether and chloroform anesthesia for general surgery in 1846. The surgical patient would inhale these anesthetic gases into the lungs, and then fall into an unconscious state. Within a few months of introducing anesthetic gases in surgical practice, physicians began to use them to relieve the pain of labor and delivery. The dream of pain-free childbirth had become a reality.

Mothers-to-be gradually embraced the idea of anesthesia for childbirth, especially after several prominent women acclaimed the procedure after having experienced it. Dr. James Young Simpson, a renowned Scottish obstetrician, was the first to give anesthesia (ether) for childbirth on January 19, 1847. Four months later in the United States, Dr. Nathan Cooley Keep, a Massachusetts dentist and physician, administered ether to Fanny Appleton Longfellow, the wife of the poet Henry Wadsworth Longfellow, for the birth of their third child. Having experienced two previous deliveries without the benefit of pain relief, Fanny Longfellow was uniquely qualified to speak on the subject. She extolled the virtues of anesthesia as "certainly the greatest blessing of this age."[3]

Six years later, in 1853, London physician Dr. John Snow anesthetized Queen Victoria with chloroform to ease the pain of delivering her seventh child, Prince Leopold. When Queen Victoria's eldest daughter gave birth in 1860, also with the benefit of anesthesia, the Queen remarked "What a blessing she had chloroform!"[4] This royal approval encouraged other Englishwomen to request similar treatment.

From the start, however, the concept of pain relief for labor was opposed as strongly as it was embraced. Some leading obstetricians of the day viewed the use of anesthesia in childbirth as an interference with the natural order of things. They argued that systemic anesthetics would harm the uterus and the progress of labor, and that inducing unconsciousness could be unsafe for the mother. There was also concern that anesthetic gases administered to the mother would cross the placenta and have detrimental effects on the newborn, making the baby sleepy and sluggish, and possibly subject to other, unknown long-term side effects. Dr. Charles D. Meigs of Philadelphia was one of the mid-19th century obstetricians who forcefully opposed pain relief for childbirth. Not very kindly, Meigs maintained "that the pain of labor had never been great enough to prevent women from having more children." [5]

Other physicians were opposed to childbirth pain relief on philosophical or religious grounds. Some based their argument against providing pain relief on the passage in Genesis 3:16 "In pain shall you bear children," which was Eve's punishment for tempting Adam with the forbidden fruit.

Physicians who became adept at administering the new anesthetics witnessed dramatic results in their patients, and their experience transformed them into passionate proponents of childbirth pain relief. Their enthusiasm for the comfort that they were able to provide outweighed the risk of any side effects they may have observed. Dr. Walter Channing, an obstetrician and dean of the Harvard Medical School from 1819 to 1847, was the leading American advocate of administering ether to women giving birth.

Social attitudes towards pain were quite complex, but during the 19th century they underwent tremendous change. The enlightened public began to praise the ability of doctors to alleviate pain: they viewed it as a human triumph over the dark forces of nature. This philosophical view, widely held in Europe and America at the time, provided a receptive audience for the argument favoring anesthesia in childbirth. Ultimately, anesthesia for childbirth gained widespread acceptance because women themselves insisted that their physicians provide pain relief. Dr. Donald Caton details this history in his excellent book, *What a Blessing She Had Chloroform: The Medical and Social Response to the Pain of Childbirth from 1800 to the Present* (Yale University Press, 1999).

Not everyone in the 19th century felt that relieving childbirth pain was desirable, and some negative attitudes toward pain relief persist today. These objections are based more on "scientific" considerations than religious ones. For example, some argue that the potential harm to the baby, the mother or the progress of labor outweighs the benefits of the epidural. Others argue against labor pain relief in the name of natural childbirth. Some natural childbirth enthusiasts believe that using pain relievers may lead to a cascade of other interventions, which could ultimately result in the use of forceps or even a cesarean delivery. I discuss these concerns in detail in Chapter Ten.

TWILIGHT SLEEP

In 1903, an alternative to ether and chloroform for relief of childbirth pain was introduced in Europe. The new systemic technique was the injection of the narcotic, morphine, combined with the amnesia-inducing drug scopolamine. Injection of these drugs resulted in a state called "twilight sleep." In this condition, the mother had no recollection of the pain of delivery, owing to the potent amnesia-producing properties of scopolamine.

A prime advantage of twilight sleep was the relative simplicity of the procedure: it was much easier to give a patient an injection than to have her inhale an anesthetic gas. But twilight sleep proved to be less than ideal for childbirth. Morphine did not relieve pain completely, while scopolamine prevented the woman from experiencing the extraordinary act of giving birth. The result was an incoherent mother with no memory of the delivery. Moreover, morphine resulted in sleepy newborns: some had significant problems breathing, while others were born asphyxiated. Despite these drawbacks, twilight sleep was very popular, and some women in the United States continued to use it as late as the 1960s.

Pregnant Pause

With twilight sleep, women were unaware of their delivery. We now know that this wasn't such a great idea. Not only did mothers miss the exciting moment of birth, but being essentially unconscious exposed them and their babies to serious medical risks as well.

DEMEROL AND OTHER NARCOTICS

Another injectable systemic narcotic, Demerol, was introduced in labor and delivery suites in the United States in 1948. Like morphine, Demerol produces more drowsiness than pain relief, and is associated with many side effects, including nausea, vomiting and itching. It may also cause a slow rate of breathing in the newborn. Despite these drawbacks, Demerol achieved immense popularity, and it is still used in many hospitals. Other injectable narcotic medications have also been used over the years to treat labor pain. One of the more popular ones has been Stadol, which is preferred by some over Demerol because it is less likely to cause slowing of breathing in the mother and newborn. However, Stadol occasionally causes feelings of anxiety, depression, restlessness and/or hallucinations.

Pregnant Pause

Narcotics such as Demerol and morphine administered systemically during labor are not very effective pain relievers and may cause many side effects in the mother-to-be such as drowsiness, nausea and vomiting, and slowing of breathing.

REGIONAL PAIN RELIEF

Local anesthetics, which block the pain message from traveling through nerves, were first used in the 1880s. It wasn't long afterward that scientists discovered injection of local anesthetic into the epidural or spinal space within the vertebral column produced profound relief of pain. The name of the these anatomical spaces are used to describe the procedures themselves, hence the common use of the terms "epidural" or "spinal" to refer to these techniques of pain relief. By the mid-20th century epidurals and spinals were being used in the labor room, so women were able to have their pain relieved yet remain awake and alert to fully experience the delivery of their baby.

EPIDURALS

The epidural space is located in the spinal column just outside the dura, a layer of tissue that surrounds the spinal fluid (Figure 3-1). The epidural space can be reached using different approaches. From the 1930s through the 1960s, anesthesiologists commonly performed epidurals by inserting a needle through the caudal portion of the vertebral column, which is

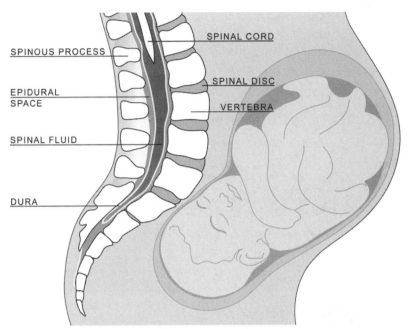

Fig. 3-1. *Side view (cross-section) of the abdomen and lower back.*

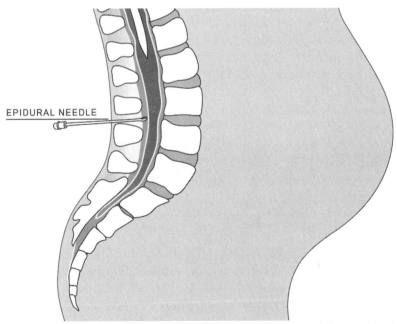

Fig. 3-2. *Side view (cross-section) of the lower portion of the vertebral column showing the epidural needle, with its tip in the epidural space.*

22

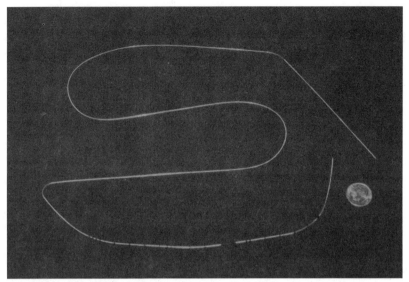

Fig. 3-3. *Epidural catheter. The dime is shown for size comparison. Only about four inches of the end of the catheter are inserted through the epidural needle into the back.*

located very low in the back, just above the coccyx (tailbone). This procedure became known as a "caudal." By the 1970s the caudal was replaced by the lumbar approach, in which the needle is placed higher up in the back (Figure 3-2). Today, nearly all labor epidurals are placed using the lumbar approach.

Once the needle tip is positioned within the epidural space, a local anesthetic may be injected. But a single dose lasts for only 20–90 minutes, depending on which anesthetic is used. The need for repeated needle insertions can be avoided by placing a catheter into the epidural space. An epidural catheter is a tiny flexible plastic tube through which the anesthetic is injected (Figure 3-3). It is very thin so it can fit through the epidural needle. After the needle tip is positioned in the epidural space, the catheter is passed through it, and the needle is removed, leaving the only the end of the catheter within the epidural space (Figure 3-4). The catheter is secured to the skin with adhesive tape. It can remain there for days, if need be (although it is hoped that labor will not last that long). Local anesthetic can then be injected through the catheter repeatedly as required, to provide pain relief for as long as is needed.

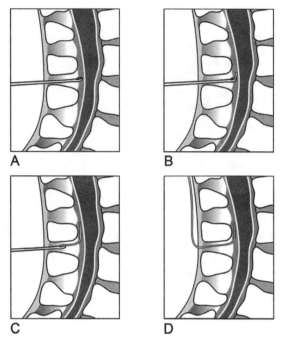

Fig. 3-4. *Insertion of an epidural catheter. A: the tip of the epidural needle is positioned within the epidural space; B: the epidural catheter is threaded through the epidural needle into the epidural space; C: the epidural needle being removed; D: the epidural needle has been completely removed, leaving only the epidural catheter within the epidural space.*

TECHNOLOGICAL ADVANCES

In the 1980s, anesthesiologists began using electronic pumps to administer the local anesthetic continuously in order to maintain the pain relief. Widely adopted during the 1990s, this practice was a great improvement because it provided a constant level of comfort instead of the "peaks and valleys" of pain and relief that had been the rule with intermittent dosing. The epidural catheter is hooked up to the pump, which is attached to a pole on wheels (the same pole on which an intravenous infusion bag is hung). This allows the woman to walk around during labor if she so desires (Figure 3-5).

An anesthesiologist practicing 50 years ago would hardly recognize the "walking epidural" (which is discussed in Chapter

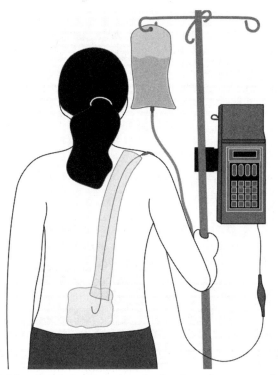

Fig. 3-5. *Epidural catheter taped to the back and connected to an infusion pump. The pump is attached to a pole on wheels — the same one on which the i.v. fluid bag hangs — allowing the woman to walk if she desires.*

Four) that is used today. The earliest epidurals produced profound muscle weakness in the legs, immobilizing the mother-to-be below the waist. However, for today's walking epidural, relatively dilute local anesthetics are used. These low-dose anesthetics cause less muscle weakness, so the woman can walk during labor if she desires and is able to push the baby out more effectively when the time comes.

Another advance is that since the early days of epidurals, new and better local anesthetics have been discovered. Also, small doses of other types of pain relievers which do not produce muscle weakness, such as synthetic narcotics, are now administered together with the local anesthetics. The result is excellent pain relief with minimal effects on muscle strength.

SPINALS

A "spinal" refers to the injection of pain-relieving medication into the spinal fluid. Unlike an epidural, the spinal needle is passed through the dura into the spinal fluid, and a single dose of medication is injected (Figure 3-6). Spinals begin to take effect much more quickly than epidurals: they work within three to five minutes as compared to ten to fifteen minutes for epidurals. But spinals don't last as long as epidurals. Spinal pain relief wears off within a few hours. This contrasts with days of pain relief that can be achieved by using an epidural catheter.

Before 1987, spinals had fallen into disfavor for childbirth because as many as 20% of women suffered a severe incapacitating headache that necessitated many days of bed rest after delivery. The problem was caused by leakage of spinal fluid through the hole that the needle made in the dura. The headache, its symptoms and its treatment is described in detail in Chapter Eight. In 1987 a major innovation in the design of the

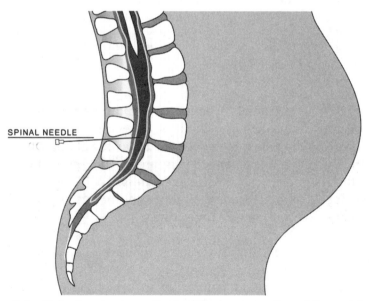

SPINAL NEEDLE

Fig. 3-6. *Side view (cross-section) of the lower portion of the vertebral column showing the spinal needle, with its tip passed through the dura into the spinal space.*

spinal needle led to a dramatic reduction in the incidence of post-spinal headache to only one to two percent of patients. The new needles had a "pencil-point" tip that produced a different shape of hole in the dura, and spinal fluid was less likely to leak through this type of hole. Pencil-point needles have made the spinal route a reasonable option for childbirth pain relief.

Pregnant Pause

One difference between a spinal and an epidural is the location where the medication is injected. With an epidural, it is injected into the epidural space, outside of the dura. With a spinal, it is injected slightly deeper (about one-quarter of an inch), through the dura and into the spinal fluid.

COMBINED SPINAL-EPIDURAL

Today, spinals and epidurals are often used interchangeably; sometimes they are even used together. With a combined spinal-epidural, the epidural needle is inserted into the epidural space, and a spinal needle is then passed through the epidural needle and through the dura to reach the spinal fluid. Anesthetic is then injected into the spinal fluid and the spinal needle is withdrawn. Next, an epidural catheter is threaded through the epidural needle, and the epidural needle is removed, leaving only the epidural catheter in place (Figure 3-7). The reasons for choosing an epidural, a spinal or a combined spinal-epidural are discussed in detail in Chapter Four.

THE MODERN ANESTHESIOLOGIST

When anesthesia was first used for childbirth 150 years ago, the specialty of anesthesiology did not yet exist. At that time, anesthetics were administered by obstetricians, dentists and others. The specialty of anesthesiology was not established until the 20th century, when residency training programs were developed. Today's anesthesiologist attends four years of medical school, followed by a year of internship and three more years of specialized training as a resident in anesthesiol-

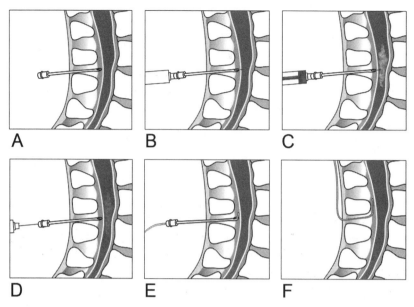

Fig. 3-7. *Combined spinal-epidural. A: epidural needle with its tip in the epidural space; B: spinal needle passed through epidural needle and through dura so that its tip rests within the spinal fluid; C: medication injected into the spinal fluid; D: spinal needle being removed; E: epidural catheter passed through epidural needle into epidural space; F: the epidural needle has been completely removed leaving only the epidural catheter within the epidural space.*

ogy. While an anesthesiologist's primary job is to provide pain relief, every anesthesiologist is also trained in resuscitation, should the need arise.

Key Concepts to Carry Away

The science and art of obstetric anesthesia has come a long way. Thanks to the new techniques of pain relief for labor and delivery that are available today, mothers-to-be may now eliminate their pain, and still be fully able to appreciate the wonder of childbirth without the suffering that their forebears were obliged to experience.

4

LEAPS AND BOUNDS:
THE WALKING EPIDURAL
AND OTHER ADVANCES

Topics Due to be Delivered

- What is a walking epidural, and how does it differ from the standard epidural?
- Medications used for low dose epidurals and spinals
- Which type of technique should you choose?
- The advantages of patient-controlled epidural analgesia

THE WALKING EPIDURAL

The primary advance made in obstetric anesthesia since I completed my training in 1986 has been the introduction of the walking epidural. The old, classic epidural numbed the lower body completely, immobilizing the woman in the process. By contrast, the walking epidural relieves the pain of labor and delivery while maintaining muscle strength, preserving the ability to walk. Aside from making walking possible, one of its distinct advantages is that it preserves pelvic and abdominal muscle tone which may be helpful in pushing the baby out during the second stage of labor. The muscle weakness produced by old-fashioned epidurals sometimes made this difficult.

It is possible to achieve the combined effects of pain relief and preserved muscle strength by using an epidural, a spinal, or a combined spinal-epidural (see Chapter Three for a detailed description of these three techniques). What matters is not the specific technique, but rather the use of a very low dose of local anesthetic.

Pregnant Pause

Many women fall asleep after getting their epidural, but it's not because medications in the epidural make them sleepy. Rather, it's because their labor pain has prevented them from sleeping—in some cases for a couple of days. Once the pain is eliminated, they are able to get some well-deserved rest so that they can save their energy for the work ahead.

The relatively high doses of local anesthetics that anesthesiologists once used compromised muscle function. Using very low concentrations of local anesthetics maintains muscle function. "But will this weak local anesthetic work?" patients often ask. The answer is yes, for most patients. Even though we now use one-half to one-tenth of the concentration previously used, we no longer depend on the local anesthetic alone: we mix other types of pain-relieving medications with it. For example, addition of a small dose of narcotic to the low dose local anesthetic is usually very effective in relieving pain. If pain persists, a higher dose of local anesthetic can easily be added.

Few women actually walk around after their pain is relieved, not because they are unable to, but because most simply prefer to rest in bed. Some women choose to take advantage of their leg strength, and may walk to the toilet in order to avoid having to use a bedpan. Others utilize their muscle strength to position themselves for delivery, for example, squatting.

THE ADVANTAGES OF COMBINING DIFFERENT TYPES OF PAIN RELIEVERS

When two different types of anesthetics are given in the epidural or spinal space at the same time, the pain relief achieved is not simply additive (1+1 = 2). Rather, the anesthetics enhance one another, as if 1+1 = 3. Also, if only small doses of each component are used, the likelihood that any individual medication will produce side effects is low. The pain relievers that anesthesiologists most commonly combine with local anesthetics are the synthetic narcotics fentanyl and sufentanil. The advantages of these medications are that they produce pain relief without causing any muscle weakness. This is because, unlike local anesthetics, narcotics administered into the spinal or epidural space block only the pain nerves, without affecting nerves that control muscle function.

The potential effect of these narcotics on babies worries more than a few mothers-to-be. But there is no need to be anxious about this. The baby is not affected by narcotics used for epidurals and spinals because the doses are so small.

EPIDURAL, SPINAL, OR COMBINED SPINAL-EPIDURAL?

Although spinals and epidurals are used almost interchangeably for childbirth, there are reasons for choosing one over the other. The main reason in deciding whether to use an epidural or a spinal has to do with timing; how long it takes for the pain relief to start working and how long it needs to last. As noted in Chapter Three, a spinal begins to work to relieve labor pain very quickly, within three to five minutes, while an epidural takes about 10 to 15 minutes to work. But spinal pain relief lasts

Pregnant Pause

Spinals begin to relieve labor pain a few minutes faster than epidurals, but don't last as long. Epidurals are much more versatile, and can provide pain relief for many hours or even days, if need be.

for only a limited time, typically less than two hours, while epidurals can be re-dosed to maintain the pain relief for as long as needed. There is a way that spinals can be made to last longer, for up to a few hours, by using a very long-lasting narcotic (morphine). In general, though, giving spinal morphine is not as reliable as giving an epidural to provide long-lasting pain relief, and it is associated with a higher likelihood of bothersome side effects such as itching, nausea, and drowsiness. Also, spinal morphine does not provide very good pain relief for the second stage of labor. The combined spinal-epidural technique has the best features of both; the spinal component begins to work rapidly and the epidural catheter can be used to give pain medication for as long as needed.

If you're in relatively early labor and still have hours to go, an epidural makes the most sense because it can last for as long as you may need it. If you don't request pain relief until the end of the first stage of labor or the beginning of the second stage, when delivery is imminent, the difference in onset time between spinals and epidurals becomes a more important factor. In such a situation, it may be advisable to use a spinal, because it will take effect very quickly and you probably won't need the pain relief to last for very long. A combined spinal-epidural may be even a better choice in this circumstance. Unlike a spinal alone, a combined spinal-epidural enables the administration of additional anesthetics through the epidural catheter, if necessary. So, if the labor is prolonged for any reason or if a cesarean is required, as much anesthesia as needed can be added.

Pregnant Pause

If you don't ask for pain relief until very late in labor, a spinal or a combined spinal-epidural are sensible choices, because medications given in the spinal fluid begin to relieve pain more quickly than medications given in the epidural space.

Some anesthesiologists advocate use of a combined spinal-epidural early in the first stage of labor. They start by giving a dose through the spinal and then they administer the epidural dose as the spinal medication begins to wear off. But if you have hours of labor ahead, I wouldn't advise having a combined spinal-epidural just to get the pain relieved five minutes faster. If your cervix is two to three centimeters dilated, and your obstetrician or midwife has determined that you are truly in labor, I would recommend a low-dose epidural. The best way to avoid a situation where it is crucial that you need the anesthetic to take effect immediately is to insert an epidural catheter early on, *before* the severe pain begins. The rationale for this approach is discussed in more detail in Chapter Five.

THE RIGHT AMOUNT

Ideally, you would receive the exact amount of anesthetic necessary to relieve your pain, no more and no less. But it is impossible at the outset to predict the precise amount of medication that any particular mother-to-be will require, because everyone has different needs, and because every labor is unique. Our approach is to start with a dose that is likely to relieve pain in most—but not necessarily all—women. We then fine-tune pain relief by giving booster doses as needed through the epidural catheter to make you comfortable, or by allowing you to self-administer booster doses (see Patient-Controlled Epidural Analgesia, below). This approach tends to prevent you from receiving more medication than you need. In general, it is easier to add more pain relievers as needed than to wait for an excess to wear off.

PATIENT-CONTROLLED EPIDURAL ANALGESIA (PCEA)

Continuous administration of pain relievers into the epidural space was made possible by electronic pumps that came into use in the 1980s. This technology has had a profound impact on the practice of obstetric anesthesia. Before these pumps were used, the anesthesiologist would have to keep giving doses of epidural pain medication every so often during labor. By continuously delivering a regulated flow of medication, the pumps have solved the problem of the pain that typically occurred between the time that one dose wore off and the next dose began to work. Once started, a pump can deliver medication for the duration of labor and delivery, maintaining constant relief with a low-dose mixture of pain relievers, usually a local anesthetic and a synthetic narcotic, as described above.

Epidural Episodes:
"DON'T GIVE HER TOO MUCH, DOC"

I was called to care for S.G., who was having her first baby. She thought that she wanted an epidural, but was unsure because she had heard a couple of frightening epidural stories. When her labor pain became very intense she decided to ask for an epidural. As I was administering the medication her husband said "Don't give her too much, Doc." His concern that the epidural could be harmful to his wife or their baby, although admirable, was misplaced. Many parents-to-be have expressed these concerns to me. I explain that they shouldn't worry, because with a walking epidural, we administer only a small amount of medication, so it's not dangerous for mother or baby.

Another technological advance was the introduction of programmable pumps that allowed women to control administration of their own pain medication by pushing a button. This can be done in two ways: by allowing the mother-to-be to get booster doses without any "background" flow of medication, or by delivering a low background flow and allowing her to fine-tune the pain control with booster doses. The technique is known as "patient-controlled epidural analgesia" (PCEA). It has a built-in safety mechanism, as the anesthesiologist sets the maximum amount of medication that the pump will administer. That way, it is not possible for the woman to overdose herself, even if she constantly pushes the button.

Pregnant Pause

Find out if patient-controlled regional analgesia (PCEA) is available at the hospital where you will be delivering.

PCEA is an excellent way to give epidural medication during labor. Studies have shown that women find this approach more satisfying than when they are not able to dose themselves. This is because they perceive themselves to be—and indeed are—more in control of their situation. Another advantage of PCEA is that women are more likely to succeed in pushing effectively during the second stage because they tend to retain the feeling of pressure as the baby descends towards the birth canal. The reason for this is that by fine-tuning their own medication, they are more likely to give themselves just enough to feel the pressure but not the pain.

Key Concepts to Carry Away

The scientific and technological advances that made walking epidurals (and spinals) possible have revolutionized obstetric anesthesia. Women are now able to be free of the pain of labor and delivery while retaining the muscle strength needed to effectively push the baby out.

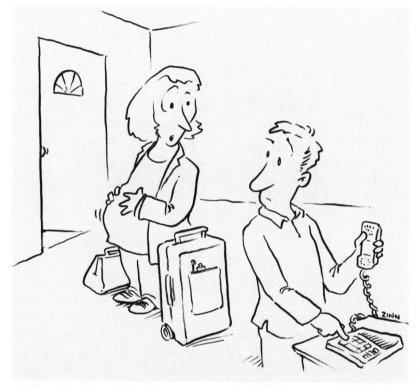

"When I said call the doctor, I meant the ANESTHESIOLOGIST! I want my epidural!"

5

THE TIMING OF LABOR PAIN RELIEF

 Topics Due to be Delivered
- **Is it ever "too early" or "too late" to get an epidural?**
- **When should you ask for pain relief?**
- **Should the pain relief be continued during the second stage of labor?**

CONFUSING MISINFORMATION

Many women suffer needlessly for hours in labor because they are led to believe that it is either "too early" or "too late" to get an epidural. The reason? The continuing prevalence of old-fashioned and outdated notions about when epidurals can and should be given. These misconceptions are widely held not only by the women themselves, but even by some obstetric caregivers—doctors, midwives and nurses alike.

Many people mistakenly believe in the "window-of-opportunity" concept of pain relief: the idea that there is a specific interval during which an epidural or spinal can be safely administered. This "window-of-opportunity" is usually believed to occur when the cervix is dilated between four and seven centimeters. The misguided thinking is that pain relief given "too early" will slow down the progress of labor and may make it necessary to use forceps in the delivery, or even to perform a cesarean. If it is given "too late," the story goes, it may impair the woman's ability to push, or may not take effect rapidly enough to be worthwhile. Neither view has a sound scientific basis.

TOO EARLY TO GET AN EPIDURAL?

The "it's too early" idea grew out of research conducted during the 1950s, when the use of regional pain relief was becoming popular. Flawed interpretation of data at that time about the effect of caudal epidurals on the course of labor resulted in the inappropriate recommendation that epidurals be withheld from women in the "early" stages of labor. This became the practice for generations of obstetrical caregivers even though the caudal epidurals of the 1950s bear little resemblance to the types of epidurals currently used. The concentrations of local anesthetic used for today's walking epidurals are one-fifth of the concentrations used for caudals 50 years ago.

Pregnant Pause

Can you imagine visiting the dentist to have a tooth drilled, but insisting on not receiving a local anesthetic until *after* the drilling has begun? Sounds absurd, right? Yet this is precisely the approach that most women use for labor pain relief. They wait until the pain becomes unbearable before they get the epidural.

DATA ABOUT EARLY EPIDURALS

In 2005, Dr. Cynthia Wong and colleagues published a landmark study of the effects of early spinal-epidurals on the progress and outcome of labor in women having their first baby.[6] Mothers-to-be who requested pain relief before their cervix was dilated to four centimeters were given either systemic (i.v. narcotics) or regional (combined spinal-epidural) pain relief. Once their cervix reached four centimeters dilation, all women were given patient-controlled epidural analgesia (PCEA; see page 33). The doctors then observed the course of labor and delivery.

Epidural Episodes:
WELCOME TO THE 21st CENTURY

P.B. was a 26-year-old first-time mother-to-be. When she visited her obstetrician in the morning, her cervix was closed. By the time P.B. arrived at the labor and delivery suite in the afternoon, her cervix had opened to two centimeters. She was walking—or attempting to walk—up and down the hall. I watched as she moved tentatively for a few feet until a contraction forced her to lean over and grab the wall railing, groaning in pain. Her devoted husband massaged her lower back through her hospital gown. I introduced myself and asked whether she had considered an epidural. I got the stock answer: it was "too early" to get one because her cervix was not dilated enough. Speaking to the young couple between her contractions, I explained that if she was in pain, it was not "too early" to get relief. I mentioned that even with an epidural or spinal, she would probably still be able to walk as much as she wanted because I would use very low doses of anesthetics, just enough to relieve her pain, but not to weaken her muscles. The prospective parents seemed at once confused, suspicious and hopeful, which was an understandably mixed reaction given what they had heard before I met them. I spoke with her obstetrician, who agreed with my plan to administer a walking epidural. In 20 minutes, she was comfortable. The husband seemed to be as pleased as his wife after she was relieved of her severe pain—the kind that women have always had to endure—to the pain-free comfort that is possible in a 21st-century labor suite.

The rate of cesarean was nearly identical whether the women received i.v. narcotics (21% cesareans) or a combined spinal-epidural (18% cesareans). Interestingly, labor progressed more rapidly if a combined spinal-epidural was given; those women reached full cervical dilation (ten centimeters) an hour-and-a-half sooner than women who received i.v. narcotics. Not surprisingly, the combined spinal-epidural provided better pain relief than did the i.v. narcotics. This study confirms what anesthesiologists have been saying for years: it's sensible to give epidurals and spinals early in labor.

PAIN AS INDICATOR OF DYSFUNCTIONAL LABOR

Labor is very painful for most women, but if it is dysfunctional, it may hurt even more. Dysfunctional labor means that the cervix dilates at a slower rate than normal, and delivery by forceps or cesarean is more likely. So with dysfunctional labor there is a combination of slow progress and more pain than usual. The three main causes of dysfunctional labor are inefficient uterine contractions, a large baby, or a small pelvis. Women who are experiencing dysfunctional labor are more likely to request and receive an epidural. But when it turns out that a forceps or cesarean delivery is needed, the epidural is blamed, even though there is no irrefutable evidence that the epidural itself had anything to do with the outcome of labor.

The link between pain and dysfunctional labor was noticed in 1989 by Dr. Michael Wuitchik, a Canadian obstetrician. He showed that intense pain very early in labor, before the cervix was dilated three centimeters, predicted the type of delivery that the women would have. Sixty-eight percent of women who reported "horrible" or "excruciating" pain during very early labor went on to have forceps or cesarean delivery. On the other hand, only 30% of women who rated their pain as only "discomforting" went on to have cesarean or forceps delivery. In other words, intense pain very early on in labor was an indicator that labor would be dysfunctional and that forceps or cesarean delivery would be more likely.[7]

Thus, the fact that a woman has pain early on in the process of labor may simply be a sign of dysfunctional labor. Refusing to relieve the pain, even before the cervix is three centimeters dilated, makes no sense.

TOO LATE FOR AN EPIDURAL?

The misconception that it may be too late to get an epidural has probably been around for as long as epidurals have been used. Since epidurals take a while to begin working, usually 10 to 15 minutes, they were not considered to be a good choice for providing pain relief for a woman rapidly approaching the moment of birth.

If anesthesia was needed quickly — for example, for a forceps delivery in a woman who didn't have an epidural catheter in place — a type of spinal anesthesia called a "saddle block" was given. It got this name because it anesthetized the area of skin that makes contact with the saddle when one rides a horse. The advantage of this type of a spinal compared to an epidural was that it worked more quickly, in about three to five minutes. However, the relatively high concentration of local anesthetic used for saddle blocks produced profound muscle weakness, making it difficult for the woman to push her baby out.

The introduction of new low-dose techniques of spinal anesthesia in the late 1980s changed all this. It became possible to administer a spinal anesthetic that would take effect within three to five minutes and at the same time preserve the muscle strength needed to push effectively. In fact, because of its rapid onset, a low-dose spinal or a combined spinal-epidural is now the procedure of choice when delivery is imminent.

WHAT'S THE OFFICIAL ACOG POSITION?

The Committee on Obstetric Practice of the American College of Obstetricians and Gynecologists (ACOG) periodically issues "Committee Opinions" to advise obstetricians of current thinking on various topics. In February 2002, ACOG published Committee Opinion #269, which took head-on the controversial practice of waiting until the cervix was dilated four to five centimeters before giving an epidural:

...[I]t has come to the attention of ACOG that some institutions are now requiring that laboring women reach four to five centimeters of cervical dilatation before receiving epidural analgesia...Labor results in severe pain for many women. There is no other circumstance where it is considered acceptable for a person to experience untreated severe pain, amenable to safe intervention, while under a physician's care. In the absence of a medical contraindication, maternal request is a sufficient medical indication for pain relief during labor.[8]

So ACOG comes squarely down on the side of labor pain relief on demand.

WHEN YOU SHOULD ASK FOR PAIN RELIEF

At what point during labor may you ask for pain relief? And at what point should you ask for relief? The answers to these questions will be different for every woman and can even vary for the same woman from one labor to the next. If you have decided in advance that you want regional pain relief, I would recommend that you have the epidural catheter inserted as soon as your obstetrician or midwife determines that you are truly in labor and will be staying in the hospital. I would also advise that you have the epidural catheter inserted even if you're not in labor, provided that your obstetric caregiver has made a decision to deliver the baby, for example, if your water has broken. You need not wait until the pain begins to have the catheter inserted. Of course, your obstetric caregiver has to be in agreement with this plan.

Pregnant Pause

You should discuss the issue of the timing of pain relief with your obstetrician or midwife during your pregnancy, so that you can agree on an approach before labor begins.

After the anesthesiologist has inserted the epidural catheter, he or she can hook the catheter to an electronic infusion pump. With the catheter in place, it is a simple matter to turn the pump on, which will then send the correct dosage of the medication into your epidural space. In this way, you will be all set to receive pain medication when you decide that you want it, assuming, of course, that your obstetrician or midwife agrees.

If you wait until you are in severe pain to have the epidural catheter inserted, you are making the situation a bit more difficult for yourself. This is because it is not as easy to remain still while the epidural is being inserted if you are in pain. Keep in mind, also, that the anesthesiologist may not be available at the precise moment you decide that you want pain relief. Consider how the labor and delivery unit in a hospital functions: there are usually many patients, all in various stages of labor. Just when your pain is becoming unbearable and minutes start to feel like hours, the anesthesiologist on duty may be busy caring for another woman, and you may have to wait. Remember, too, that an epidural takes 10 to 15 minutes to work once the medication is injected into the catheter. By far the most sensible option is to have the epidural catheter inserted early, before the severe pain begins.

Pregnant Pause

If you have decided that you are definitely going to want an epidural, then request to have the epidural catheter inserted when you are admitted to the hospital, assuming that it has been established that you are truly in labor. In this way, as soon as you decide you want the pain relief started, it will be a simple matter to inject the medication through the catheter into your epidural space.

IS IT EVER TOO LATE FOR EPIDURAL OR SPINAL PAIN RELIEF?

No, it is never too late for pain relief. I have administered epidurals and spinals to many women who were dilated to eight, nine or even ten centimeters and were about to begin the second stage of labor (pushing). Patients who receive pain relief in this situation have been very appreciative to have been spared the pain of late labor and delivery. Afterward, many have wondered aloud why they had not opted for it earlier.

Epidural Episodes:
BETTER LATE THAN NEVER

J.S. was having her second baby. She had delivered her first baby vaginally, without an epidural, and she was planning to do it the same way this time as well. She bore the pain as her cervix dilated, but when it reached ten centimeters, the trouble began. The baby was not descending properly and because of her intense pain, she was not able to push effectively. Her obstetrician recommended that she assume a squatting position to assist the baby's descent, but her pain prevented her from doing even that. The obstetrician requested that I administer pain relief that would allow effective pushing. I gave J.S. a low-dose spinal. This provided rapid pain relief and preserved her muscle strength so that she could squat and push well. Within an hour she had delivered a beautiful baby. After it was over, her obstetrician remarked that without the spinal, he would have had to perform a cesarean.

The important point here is that it is not unreasonable to ask for pain relief even if you are dilated to ten centimeters. If delivery is expected to occur within a few minutes it probably is not worthwhile. On the other hand, if the pushing stage lasts for a long time, a spinal and/or epidural can be enormously beneficial. For women having their first baby, this may be two or three hours, or more. There is no way of predicting precisely how long your second stage will last, although your obstetrician or midwife will be able to give you an educated guess. While I am not recommending that you wait until full dilation to ask for it, keep in mind that just because you're far along, doesn't mean that you can't have pain relief.

KEEPING THE EPIDURAL GOING THROUGH DELIVERY

Another important issue about the timing of pain relief is how long to keep it going. Many people are still under the impression that the epidural must be turned off or at least dialed down for the delivery. In some cases, this may be true. If you can't sense any pressure during the second stage as the baby descends, pushing is difficult. It is certainly easier to push against something, than just to push in the abstract. Ideally, the epidural (or spinal) will take away the pain sensation but leave you with a sensation of pressure. If you can't feel any pressure sensation at all, then your epidural medication may have to be decreased. As the pain relief begins to wear off, the pressure sensation will return. It's best to begin pushing as you begin to sense the pressure, before the severe pain returns. We have found that using patient-controlled epidural analgesia (PCEA) tends to preserve the pressure sensation, because women in labor give themselves just enough pain medication to take the pain away without abolishing the pressure sensation that accompanies each contraction.

Key Concepts to Carry Away

A woman should receive pain relief when she wants it. She should not have to wait until someone else deems it permissible. Consider a commonsense approach to pain relief. Childbirth hurts, but you can dramatically diminish and perhaps even eliminate the pain by choosing to use a regional pain relief technique. Ideally, you should have the epidural and/or spinal in place before the severe pain starts, so long as labor has been diagnosed, or a decision has been made to deliver the baby. The pain relief should be continued through delivery.

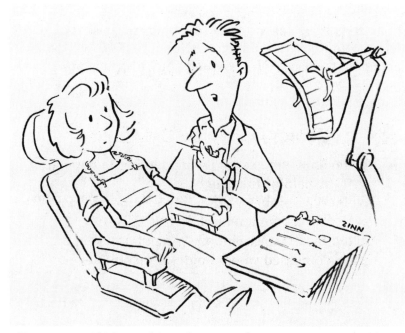

"Let me see if I have this right—you don't want me to give you the local anesthesia until **after** I've started the drilling?"

6

EPIDURALS AND SPINALS:
A GUIDED TOUR

Topics Due to be Delivered

- **Knowing exactly what is going to happen is helpful to reduce anxiety**
- **Why proper positioning is important for a successful epidural and/or spinal**
- **Step-by-step descriptions of epidural, spinal, and combined spinal-epidural techniques**

ANTICIPATION

What can you expect to happen as your anesthesiologist administers your epidural or spinal? Knowing what is coming will help to allay any concerns you may have. While the prospect of a needle being inserted into your back is hardly pleasant, perception truly is worse than the reality. Keep in mind that the actual insertion is quick, and that a local anesthetic is used to numb the area beforehand. And remember that the epidural and spinal needles are in place for only a minute or two—just long enough to insert a tiny flexible plastic catheter into the epidural space or to inject medication into the spinal fluid.

MONITORING

Before you receive your epidural and/or spinal, as many as three devices will be put into position to allow the anesthesiologist to monitor your vital signs. A blood pressure cuff will be placed around your upper arm. Today, these cuffs are automatic — a machine has replaced the stethoscope. The first time that the device takes your blood pressure, the cuff squeezes your arm very tightly. Electrocardiogram (EKG) leads may be attached to your chest and shoulders by small adhesive patches to monitor your heart function. Third, a pulse oximeter, which resembles a cushioned clothespin, may be placed on one of your fingertips to measure the amount of oxygen in your blood. Your baby's heart rate will also be monitored.

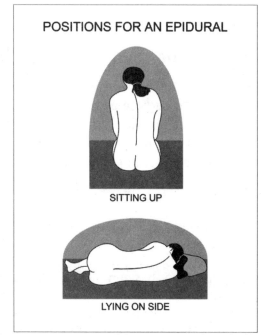

Fig. 6-1. *The two positions used for insertion of epidurals and spinals.*

POSITIONING IS IMPORTANT

Next, to make your epidural and/or spinal space as accessible as possible for the anesthesiologist, you will be positioned in one of two ways, either sitting or lying on your side (Figure 6-1). The purpose of both positions is the same: to help you round out your lower back as much as possible. This outwardly-curled position of your lower back increases the opening between the spinous processes, the little bumps you can feel running down the center of your back. This is important as it is much easier for your anesthesiologist to direct the epidural and/or spinal needle to the desired location when these spaces are widened (Figure 6-2). If you are in a sitting position, you will be asked to dangle your arms in front of you, which relaxes your shoulders forward and helps you push your lower back out. If you are lying on your side, you will be asked to curl into a fetal position. Do your best, but in either position, we understand that it's challenging to curl up and bring your knees to your chest with a pregnant abdomen in the way.

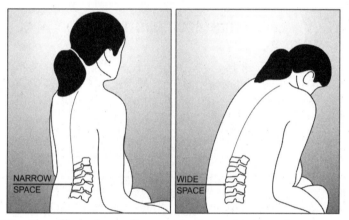

Fig. 6-2. *The effect of rounding out the lower back on the space between the spinous processes. Note how the distance between the spinous processes widens when the back is rounded out. This is important as the epidural and/or spinal needle must pass between the spinous processes (see also Figure 3-1).*

CLEANING AND NUMBING

Once you are in position, your back will be cleansed with an antiseptic solution such as Betadine. Because this solution is at room temperature, it feels cold when it is applied to your skin. After your skin has been cleansed, the anesthesiologist will place a drape over your back. The drape has a hole in it, to allow access to the area where the epidural and/or spinal needle will be inserted.

Just before the anesthesiologist inserts the epidural and/or spinal needle, he or she will numb a small area of skin by injecting a local anesthetic. Most women later tell me that the skin numbing was the only painful part of the entire epidural or spinal procedure and that it hurt less than having the i.v. inserted.

Pregnant Pause

I explain that getting an epidural and/or a spinal is about as painful as having an i.v. inserted. After I finish, most women tell me that their i.v. hurt more.

FINALLY—YOU'RE READY FOR THE EPIDURAL AND/OR SPINAL

After your skin has been numbed with local anesthetic, you should feel a sensation of pressure—but not pain—when the epidural and/or spinal needle is inserted. If you do sense any pain, tell your anesthesiologist so that he or she can give you more local anesthetic before proceeding further. The anesthesiologist depends on feedback from you for guidance. By the same token, your anesthesiologist should explain every step of the procedure so that you are not surprised by anything that occurs. Next comes the most demanding part of the procedure for your anesthesiologist—the actual insertion of the tip of the needle into the epidural or spinal space. The technique is based on feel since it is not possible to see the epidural or spinal space —and skill attained through experience.

For an epidural, once the needle tip is in position, a tiny catheter is threaded through it into the epidural space. The catheter is a thin, flexible tube with one to three holes at its tip through which anesthetic medication is injected into the epidural space. If it brushes against a nerve root as it passes in, you may experience a "funny-bone" sensation in your back, hip or leg. Although this is uncomfortable, it passes quickly, and there is no cause for alarm. With the newer, more flexible epidural catheters, the likelihood of experiencing this sensation has been reduced.

After the epidural catheter is inserted, your anesthesiologist will remove the needle, leaving a couple of inches of catheter within your epidural space. Then he or she will secure the catheter to your back with adhesive tape. Having an epidural catheter in place will not prevent you from lying on your back or moving around. You do not have to worry about its becoming dislodged unintentionally. Although this may occur, it is unlikely. The adhesive tape is so sticky that patients say removing it reminds them of a skin waxing. For a spinal, once the needle is inserted, anesthetic medication will be injected into the spinal fluid and then the needle will be removed.

If you are given a combined spinal-epidural, the epidural needle is first placed in the epidural space, and then a spinal needle is passed through the epidural needle and through the dura to reach the spinal fluid. After the anesthetic medication is injected, the spinal needle is withdrawn and a catheter is threaded through the epidural needle into the epidural space. The epidural needle is then withdrawn and the catheter is secured to your back with adhesive tape, as described above. Having worked with thousands of patients, and having undergone spinal anesthesia myself, I can assure you that the procedure really isn't very painful.

Key Concepts to Carry Away

Keep an open mind about your pain relief options. Usually, the thought of getting an epidural or spinal is much worse than the procedure itself. For most women, the insertion of an epidural or spinal hurts a lot less than does a uterine contraction.

7

IF YOUR DELIVERY IS CESAREAN

Topics Due to be Delivered

- The difference between planned, urgent, and emergency cesareans
- Anesthetic choices for cesarean
- Why regional anesthesia is preferred for cesarean
- The risks of general anesthesia
- A detailed description of what will occur in the operating room
- The importance of remaining focused on the big picture

PLANNED, URGENT AND EMERGENCY CESAREANS

More than one out of every four babies in the United States is born by cesarean delivery, and if the current trend continues, soon it will be one out of every three. Some cesareans are planned long before labor actually begins. Unplanned cesareans, decided upon once labor is under way, have different degrees of urgency. For example, if a baby is discovered to be in the breech position rather than headfirst, a cesarean may be called for, but the situation is not necessarily an emergency. However, if the fetal heart rate slows and does not recover, an extremely urgent or "stat" cesarean is called for (from *statim*, the Latin word for "immediately"). The type of anesthesia that is chosen is largely determined by the urgency of the situation.

GENERAL VERSUS REGIONAL ANESTHESIA

Today, more than 90% of planned cesareans in the United States are performed using regional anesthesia (epidurals and spinals). Until the 1970s–1980s, general anesthesia was the technique of choice for cesarean delivery in hospitals nation-wide. Its use began to decline as its drawbacks for baby and mother became increasingly clear:

- The general anesthetics that produce unconsciousness in the mother pass through the placenta and may also cause the baby to be born sleepy and breathing too slowly. If this occurs, the newborn may require assistance breathing until the effects of the general anesthetics wear off.

- For general anesthesia, a breathing tube must be inserted into the trachea (windpipe); this is known as intu-

Epidural Episodes:

IN A FLASH

A.F. was in labor with her first baby. She was not sure that she wanted an epidural, and was using breathing techniques to deal with the pain of her contractions. Her cervix was dilated five centimeters when her nurse noticed that the baby's heart rate was slowing. It had been 130 to 140 beats per minute, but it was now 70 to 80 beats per minute, and wasn't improving. Her obstetrician was notified immediately, and he decided to quickly bring A.F. to the cesarean section room. I was paged stat and while her bed was being rolled down the hall, I assured A.F. that we would do our very best to see that she and her baby would be fine. I gave her general anesthesia and three minutes later her obstetrician delivered the baby. Fortunately, mother and baby did very well and they both went home four days later. General anesthesia was key in this case, as it made possible rapid delivery of the baby.

bation. During this procedure it is possible that residual food or liquid in the stomach can be vomited and spilled into the lungs. This is known as aspiration, and doesn't happen with regional anesthesia, because when we're awake, our gag reflex protects us.

- With general anesthesia the mother is not awake to enjoy the birth of her baby.

On the other hand, it is important to bear in mind that except in rare cases, general anesthesia is a safe, reliable method for women who want or need it. The pediatrician can help the newborn breathe if necessary, and the anesthesiologist will maximize the chance of a successful intubation, and minimize the chance that aspiration will occur. In some situations, general anesthesia may be the only option. Regional anesthesia cannot be used if:

- The baby has a dangerously slow heart rate and a stat cesarean delivery becomes necessary, with no time to spare. In most cases, it takes less time to give general anesthesia than to give an epidural or spinal. However, in some circumstances — for example, if an epidural catheter is already in place and being used to provide labor pain relief — it is a simple matter for the anesthesiologist to inject additional medication through the catheter, allowing the obstetrician to proceed with the cesarean.

- The mother-to-be has substantial bleeding that causes her blood pressure to fall. Since the doses of anesthetics used for cesareans done under epidurals and spinals have a tendency to lower blood pressure, general anesthesia is probably a better choice in this circumstance.

- There is a skin infection on the lower back. The needle could transport bacteria from the skin into the epidural or spinal space, causing a serious infection such as meningitis.

- There is a bleeding disorder. If the blood does not clot normally, and the epidural or spinal needle nicks a vein, excessive bleeding may occur in the epidural or spinal space. This could cause permanent damage to nerves in the area if the problem is not recognized and quickly corrected.

- If the mother-to-be refuses to have a needle inserted into her back.

Pregnant Pause

There are certain circumstances when general anesthesia may be necessary for cesarean. Although regional anesthesia is usually preferable, don't worry if you need general anesthesia. It has been used for many years and has an excellent success rate.

DIFFERENCES BETWEEN REGIONAL PAIN RELIEF FOR LABOR AND REGIONAL ANESTHESIA FOR CESAREANS

The dose of local anesthetic required for spinals and epidurals for cesareans is much higher than the dose required for relieving the pain of labor. This higher anesthetic concentration will make you feel very numb, and because it affects muscle function, you should expect your legs to be weak. In fact, you may not be able to move your legs at all for a few hours after the operation. Some women are concerned by this loss of muscle function. But there is no need to worry, as this is expected, temporary and not dangerous.

WHICH WILL IT BE: SPINAL OR EPIDURAL?

If you receive regional anesthesia for your cesarean, which will it be: spinal, epidural or a combined spinal-epidural? If you happen to have an epidural catheter already in place for labor, then your anesthesiologist will continue with the epidural by simply injecting a higher dose of local anesthetic through the catheter. If your cesarean is planned, most anesthesiologists in the United States prefer to use a spinal. Some may prefer to use an epidural, and others will use a combined spinal-epidural technique. As discussed in Chapter Two, each technique has its advantages and disadvantages, and there is no one "right way." The spinal takes effect more rapidly than does an epidural. While this may not make a difference for a planned cesarean, for an urgent or emergency cesarean, saving a few minutes may be important. However, a spinal lasts only as long as a single dose works. Epidurals can be made to last indefinitely, because extra doses of medication can be injected through the catheter as needed. Furthermore, the epidural catheter may be left in place to provide pain relief after the cesarean (see Chapter Nine). A combined spinal-epidural technique has both advantages – the anesthesia takes effect rapidly and there is an option to give additional doses of anesthetics, if necessary.

Pregnant Pause

Cesareans may be performed under spinal, epidural, or combined spinal-epidural anesthesia. All of these options provide excellent pain relief for the surgery.

A STEP-BY-STEP TOUR OF THE CESAREAN EXPERIENCE

Knowing what will happen will help to make the experience less intimidating. When you are brought into the operating room, you will probably immediately notice that the room is very cold. In fact, it is common hospital practice to keep operating rooms cold so that the surgeons, who wear surgical gowns over their scrub suits, will be comfortable. The problem is that, as the patient, you are wearing only a thin hospital gown with an embarrassingly open back. Short of insisting that the entire operating room be warmed—which may not be such a bad idea—you can ask to be covered with warm blankets (except for your abdomen of course, where the incision will be made).

After you are positioned on the operating table, monitoring devices (discussed in Chapter Six) will be put into place, including a blood pressure cuff around your arm, EKG leads on your chest and shoulders, and a pulse oximeter on your finger. Your anesthesiologist will use these devices throughout the cesarean to monitor your vital signs (blood pressure, pulse, heart rhythm and the amount of oxygen in your blood).

IF YOU RECEIVE GENERAL ANESTHESIA

If you are to receive general anesthesia, an oxygen mask will be placed over your nose and mouth. You will be instructed to take some deep breaths to fill your lungs completely with pure oxygen before going to sleep. Anesthetics will then be administered through your i.v. line to rapidly make you sleepy. Once you are asleep, the anesthesiologist will place a breathing tube in your trachea (windpipe). This tube is used to provide oxygen and anesthetic gases during the operation. As soon as the cesarean is completed, the anesthesiologist will awaken you and immediately remove the breathing tube. Very few people have any recollection of the breathing tube at all; the only indication that it was there may be a mildly sore throat for a day or so.

IF YOU RECEIVE REGIONAL ANESTHESIA

If regional anesthesia is used, you will be positioned for the insertion of an epidural and/or a spinal in your lower back (see Chapter Six)—unless an epidural catheter was already placed for labor. A drop in blood pressure, which is unlikely with the low dosage of medication used for labor, can occur with the higher dose used for cesareans. Your anesthesiologist is well aware of this, and will be ready to promptly treat any fall in blood pressure with intravenous fluids and medications. Do not be surprised if you experience a temporary feeling of light-headedness or nausea as your body adapts to the anesthetic.

Before the cesarean actually begins, the obstetrician will hang a surgical drape between your chest and abdomen. This drape will prevent you from watching the operation being performed. You will probably be given oxygen to breathe through either a clear mask or plastic prongs positioned in your nostrils. This is done to provide your baby with some extra oxygen in the moments before delivery.

Before your surgery starts, your anesthesiologist will test you to ensure that the anesthesia is working properly and that you are numb. Do not be surprised if you feel a sensation of pressure during this test; this is normal. Local anesthetics block the sensation of pain, but not sensations of pressure. The sensation you will feel during the cesarean is similar to what you feel while having a tooth drilled at the dentist's office. After the dentist numbs your tooth with local anesthetic, you do not feel pain from the drilling, but you can still feel some pressure on your teeth and gums. Likewise, during the cesarean, you will feel pressure in different parts of your abdomen and chest. If the pressure sensation bothers you, or if you feel any pain, tell your anesthesiologist so that he or she can administer additional medication to make you comfortable.

Pregnant Pause

Many women are frightened that the anesthesia won't work and that they will feel the surgery. Don't worry. Before the cesarean starts your abdomen will be tested to be sure that it is completely numb.

Your arms will be placed out of the way, so that they do not interfere with the surgery. Most commonly, they are positioned on two armrests which are attached to either side of the operating table. It is important that you resist any temptation to touch your abdomen during the surgery, as this would contaminate the sterile area. Some anesthesiologists wrap adhesive tape loosely around the mothers' arms as a reminder to keep them on the armrests. Before your cesarean is started, your obstetrician will check your abdomen once again to make sure that you are completely numb. Your obstetrician will begin the cesarean only after confirming that the anesthesia is working well.

THE BIRTH

In most hospitals, when regional anesthesia is used, the spouse or partner is seated at the head of the operating table to provide support and to share in the experience of the birth. By contrast, during general anesthesia, it is the policy of most hospitals that only the surgical team be present in the room. One of the reasons for this is that the support person's assistance is of no benefit with the mother unconscious under general anesthesia. Furthermore, the presence of a non-medical person may make it more difficult for everyone to focus on his or her job, which is caring for the anesthetized mother and the newborn.

Your baby will be born within a few minutes after the beginning of the cesarean operation. If you have regional anesthesia, your obstetrician may give you a quick glimpse of your baby as soon as he or she is born. Your baby will then be cleaned up and examined. Once this is done, your baby will be wrapped in a blanket so that you and your partner can begin bonding with the baby. If you have general anesthesia, you will first meet your baby when you are awakened, as soon as the cesarean is completed.

AFTER THE BIRTH

After your baby is born, the obstetrician will close your incision in layers, working from the uterus to the skin. During this interval, some women are greatly aided by a mild sedative such as midazolam (Versed), which makes it easier to remain relaxed while the operation is completed.

REALITY CHECK: IF YOU NEED A CESAREAN

Twenty-five percent of all babies in the United States are delivered by cesarean, and that number is steadily rising, so it should not surprise you if you end up with a cesarean despite your plans to the contrary. Over the years, I have noticed that many women who were planning to deliver vaginally feel as though they have somehow failed if they need a cesarean. Their perception of failure is a result of bias that leads women to believe that vaginal delivery is good and that cesarean delivery is bad. Attitudes among women and obstetricians on this subject are changing, and cesareans by choice are gaining acceptance. In any case, it's important to keep in mind that a cesarean is just another way to have a baby, not a "worse" way.

Key Concepts to Carry Away

Modern anesthesia has helped to make cesarean delivery a comfortable, exciting and fulfilling experience. Understanding your anesthetic options for cesarean will make the entire process less intimidating.

8

THE RISKS OF REGIONAL PAIN RELIEF — AND THE RISKS OF NOT USING IT

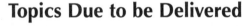

Topics Due to be Delivered

- **Headaches after epidurals and spinals**
- **Low blood pressure caused by epidurals and spinals**
- **Effects of epidurals and spinals on the baby's heart rate**
- **Rare side effects of epidurals and spinals**
- **The consequences of unrelieved pain**
- **How epidurals and spinals prevent the consequences of unrelieved pain**

CONSIDER THE RISKS AND BENEFITS

For the overwhelming majority of patients, epidurals and spinals are safe for both mother and baby. But there are risks associated with all medical procedures, and regional pain relief is no exception. No procedure is 100% guaranteed. Problems can and do occur occasionally, and epidurals and spinals may result in complications that may have short-term or (rarely) long-lasting after-effects. You need to understand the risks and benefits involved so that you can make an informed decision about using regional pain relief.

Pregnant Pause

Epidurals and spinals offer many benefits and are relatively safe procedures, but it's possible that complications may occur. You should have a thorough understanding of their benefits as well as their risks so that you can make an informed choice about what is right for you.

Keep in mind that some side effects are much more common than others, that the common ones can be dealt with easily, and that they do not have long-lasting effects. Serious side effects are rare. Finally, avoiding regional pain relief for childbirth is also associated with some risks (see below). Your anesthesiologist will discuss the risks and benefits of regional pain relief before performing the epidural or spinal, but it is difficult to concentrate on these important issues when you are experiencing labor pain. It is much better to consider the risks and benefits of regional analgesia long before your labor begins.

Risks of Regional Pain Relief

RISK: SORENESS AT THE SITE OF INSERTION

One of the most common complaints about epidurals and spinals after delivery is soreness or tenderness in the lower back at the place where the needle was inserted. The soreness is similar to a bruise, like the pain you feel after you hit your shin on a piece of furniture. The discomfort usually fades away in a couple of days. It may be treated with Tylenol. Some patients find that a heating pad is also helpful. Most women do not even notice this discomfort. They simply may not have it, or other aches and pains may be bothering them more, such as soreness of the perineum, or breast engorgement.

RISK: SPINAL HEADACHE

Headaches that are caused by either epidurals or spinals are collectively known as spinal headaches or post-dural puncture headaches. The terms are synonymous. Although headache is the most common complication of epidurals and spinals, keep in mind the chance of getting one is approximately one to two percent. While a spinal headache can be quite painful, the good news is that it can be treated. To understand the treatment, you first have to understand what causes the headache.

Spinal headaches are caused by leakage of spinal fluid through the hole in the dura that is created by the epidural or spinal needle. The spinal fluid is a clear liquid that surrounds the brain and spinal cord, and the fluid is kept in place by a layer of tissue, the dura (Figure 3-1). When a needle creates a hole in dura, the fluid may leak out, and a headache may result.

Pregnant Pause
The chance of getting a headache as a result of an epidural or spinal is small — about one or two percent. Although the headache can be very painful, don't worry, it can be treated. Just inform your anesthesiologist so that he or she can take care of your headache.

Why is the chance of getting a headache so low? The likelihood of developing a headache is directly related to the size of the hole in the dura. With an epidural, there is usually no hole at all, as your anesthesiologist makes every attempt to avoid puncturing the dura with the needle. Despite his or her best efforts, however, it still happens approximately one to two percent of the time. Since the diameter of the epidural needle is relatively large (to allow passage of the epidural catheter), the hole it creates in the dura is also relatively large, and usually results in a headache.

For spinal techniques, your anesthesiologist will intentionally pass the needle through the dura, so there is no avoiding creating a hole. However, because the spinal needle has a very small diameter—it only has to accommodate an injection of liquid medication, not a catheter—the hole made in the dura is relatively small, and is not likely to produce a headache. That's why the incidence of headache following spinal techniques is about one to two percent. Another reason for the low headache incidence has to do with the pencil-point shape of the spinal needle tips that have been in use since the mid-1980s (see Chapter 3). The actual size of the diameters of epidural and spinal needles are shown in Figure 8-1.

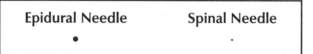

Epidural Needle   **Spinal Needle**

Fig. 8-1. *Actual size of the diameters of epidural and spinal needles shown in cross-section.*

Spinal headaches range from mild to severe. The pain may be located in the front, back, or side of the head. A mild headache may be bothersome but a severe headache may prevent you from going about your normal routine.

Spinal headaches are always worsened when you sit or stand, and tend to intensify the longer you hold your head upright. This is a unique feature of spinal headaches—they are related to your position. Lying down relieves the headache almost immediately. If the pain does not change with your position, the headache is likely to be due to some cause other than the epidural or spinal.

Pregnant Pause

Post-dural puncture (spinal) headaches are made worse by sitting upright or standing; they are relieved by lying down. If your headache does not go away when you lie down, it is highly unlikely that the epidural or spinal was the cause.

Left untreated, spinal headaches are likely to disappear on their own within one to two weeks as the hole in the dura heals. If the headache is mild and the mother has assistance at home for a few days, enabling her to spend a good amount of time resting in bed, I usually recommend a wait-and-see approach. For most women, however, this is not the case. Usually, they have to run around to care for their newborn and, possibly, older children. In this situation, the mother needs treatment quickly. If she cannot remain in bed, or if the headache is severe, I recommend an epidural blood patch.

TREATMENT OF SPINAL HEADACHE: THE EPIDURAL BLOOD PATCH

To perform an epidural blood patch, the anesthesiologist draws approximately half-an-ounce of blood from a vein in the arm and injects it into the epidural space. The blood forms a clot, which acts as a patch to plug the hole in the dura. The blood patch prevents spinal fluid from leaking out, and this relieves the symptoms of the headache (figure 8-2). Eventually, the blood clot dissolves, but by that time, your dura will have healed, closing the hole. For nearly all patients, the headache goes away as soon as the blood is injected.

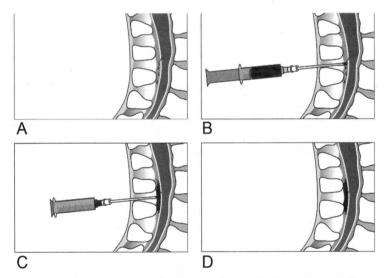

Fig. 8-2. *Epidural Blood Patch.* **A**: *spinal fluid leaking through hole in dura;* **B**: *epidural needle tip positioned in epidural space with patient's own blood in attached syringe;* **C**: *blood being injected into epidural space;* **D**: *blood in epidural space forming clot over hole in dura, preventing further leakage of spinal fluid.*

Although the epidural blood patch works immediately in nearly everyone, for approximately one in four patients, the headache returns in a day or two. This is probably caused by the blood clot "slipping" out of position so that it no longer is plugging the hole in the dura. If this happens, a second blood patch may be done. Some patients choose this option, but others may not want it since, by then, they are one day closer to the dura having healed itself.

RISK: LOW BLOOD PRESSURE

Local anesthetics injected into the epidural or spinal space may lower the mother's blood pressure. A slight decrease in pressure is not a problem. In fact, blood pressure after an epidural is generally closer to what it was before labor started, because when you're in pain, your blood pressure rises. But blood pressure that is too low can cause problems. You may feel light-headed or nauseated. More importantly, the lowered blood pressure may reduce the blood flow to the placenta, which in turn reduces the amount of oxygen that is delivered to the baby. The old-fashioned high-dose epidurals used during labor were known for causing the mother's blood pressure to fall. Anesthesiologists routinely gave fluids to the mother through her i.v. before administering the epidural to counter this anticipated effect. If the blood pressure fell despite this precaution, it was treated by giving more intravenous fluids and administering medications that increase the blood pressure. This is still done for the higher dose epidurals and spinals that are used to provide anesthesia for cesareans.

Unlike high-dose epidural and spinals, currently used low-dose walking epidurals and spinals do not usually produce a significant fall in the mother's blood pressure. This is because the low-dose methods take effect relatively slowly — over 10 to 15 minutes — giving the body time to adapt, and minimizing any effect on blood pressure. In fact, with the low dosage of epidural medication for labor used today, many anesthesiologists no longer give large amounts of intravenous fluid before the epidural. Avoiding administering this fluid has some advantages. Giving intravenous fluids before an epidural takes time. I recall many patients in the "old days" who were in severe pain but whose epidurals were delayed because they had not yet received "enough" intravenous fluid. Also, a lot of the fluid that is given through the i.v. ends up in the bladder, producing a need to urinate.

Pregnant Pause

Low blood pressure may be a problem if it reduces the blood flow (and therefore oxygen supply) to the baby. The low-dose epidurals and spinals used for labor today are unlikely to decrease blood pressure, but just in case, after you get your epidural or spinal, your blood pressure will be checked frequently, and your baby's heart rate will be monitored continuously. Should a fall in your blood pressure occur, it can be rapidly corrected.

EFFECT OF THE MOTHER'S POSITION ON BLOOD PRESSURE

Whether or not an epidural or spinal is in place, pregnant women may experience low blood pressure when they lie flat on their backs. The fall in blood pressure may cause them to feel lightheaded, flushed and shaky. This circumstance, known as the "supine hypotensive syndrome" may occur when the baby becomes heavy enough to compress two of the mother's major blood vessels, the aorta and the vena cava. These large vessels are located next to the spinal column. When they are compressed, blood flow is temporarily blocked, which causes the blood pressure to fall. Thus, it is a good idea not to lie flat on your back, but rather, to stay tilted to one side.

RISK: SPINALS, EPIDURALS AND SLOWING OF THE BABY'S HEART RATE

It is normal for the baby's heart rate to speed up and slow down during the course of labor, whether or not the mother has received regional pain relief. It is also possible that an epidural or spinal itself may cause the baby's heart rate to slow (brady-cardia). There are two ways this may happen. One is if the epidural or spinal does indeed lower the blood pressure (see discussion on blood pressure above), as low blood pressure in the mother may cause the baby's heart rate to slow. The second has nothing to do with the blood pressure, but happens some-times after spinal narcotics are given. Your anesthesiologist is aware of these possibilities, and your baby's heart rate will be closely monitored. If it slows down, your anesthesiologist will treat it by administering i.v. fluids and medications as needed.

RISK: INABILITY TO URINATE

Epidurals and spinals may numb the nerves of the bladder. If this happens, the laboring woman may not sense that her blad-der is full. Sitting on the toilet, which is possible with a walk-ing epidural, may enable her to urinate. In other cases, a uri-nary catheter may need to be inserted into her bladder to drain the urine. Bladder sensation returns as the epidural wears off. As the baby descends towards the birth canal, it sometimes blocks the flow of urine, so that bladder catheterization may be required even in women without epidurals.

RISK: PAIN DESPITE AN EPIDURAL

Sometimes women continue to feel labor pain even after receiv-ing an epidural. Should this happen to you, your anesthesiolo-gist will try to make you comfortable. There are several reasons why labor may still hurt after you get an epidural. One is sim-ply that the dose of pain medication you received was not strong enough. Each labor is different, which is why your anes-thesiologist will individualize your treatment and give you just what you need—ideally, no more and no less. One of the advantages of patient-controlled epidural analgesia (PCEA) is that you can control the amount of pain relief that you get (see Chapter Four).

Another reason that you may still have pain after receiving the epidural may be related to the position of your baby. For example, if the baby's face is looking in the direction of the ceiling (occiput posterior), labor tends to be more painful, especially in your lower back. Also, if the baby happens to be pressing directly on a nerve (or nerves) in your pelvis, it can be very painful, even with an epidural. Another cause for pain despite having an epidural is rapid progression of your labor. The more labor advances, the more it hurts. If your labor is moving very quickly, the medication you have received may not be enough to alleviate the more intense pain and you may need a booster dose of a stronger pain reliever. This is another reason for getting the epidural at an early stage. It is easier to get control of the pain before it is excruciating, and then to add stronger anesthetics as needed.

Another problem that sometimes occurs after the epidural is given is that the pain is only relieved on one side of the body. There is usually a simple explanation for this—the tip of the epidural catheter is too far over to one side. When the epidural catheter is inserted into your back, the chance of it staying exactly in the center of your epidural space is very small: it nearly always ends up on one side or the other. This situation can be corrected by pulling the catheter out a bit, a maneuver which tends to bring the tip closer to the center. This should then produce equal pain relief on both sides of the body (Figure 8-3).

Another explanation for continued pain on only one side is gravity. If you remain in one position—for example, lying on your left side for a couple of hours—gravity tends to cause the medication in your epidural space to settle on the left side. You may then feel pain on your right side. This problem can be corrected—or prevented—by changing your position and switching from lying on your right side to your left side every so often. One cause to consider for an epidural that is working well but then stops working is that the catheter may have become dislodged, so that the tip is no longer in the epidural space. This happens occasionally, and when it does, the catheter needs to be re-inserted.

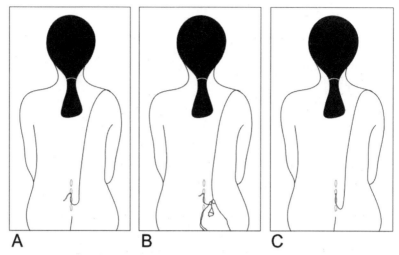

Fig. 8-3. *One-sided pain relief due to epidural catheter tip location. A: catheter tip located too far to the woman's left side; B: catheter being withdrawn slightly; C: catheter tip now located in middle.*

PUTTING THE RISK IN PERSPECTIVE

It is important to keep the risks in perspective. Most likely, you've never had an epidural or spinal before, so it is understandable if you're concerned. The overwhelming majority of women who receive regional pain relief for childbirth do not end up with any complications. For a very few, however, complications do occur. Most of these cause only temporary problems, but some rare complications are associated with long-lasting problems. So even though it's very unlikely that a serious complication will occur, it is important to understand the potential risks.

RARE RISKS OF EPIDURALS AND SPINALS

The rare complications that may occur with epidurals and spinals can be classified into two categories: local and systemic. Local complications refer to problems that are near the area where the epidural or spinal are located, and include infection, bleeding and nerve damage. Infection and bleeding are always possible when a needle is inserted anywhere in the body, and could potentially result in nerve damage or even paralysis if they are not diagnosed in time. Nerves may also be injured by the needle or catheter or due to a reaction to the medication injected. Systemic complications, which can occur if the anesthesia is unintentionally injected into the bloodstream, include seizure or even death. Unintentional injection of a high dose of anesthetic meant for the epidural space into the spinal space may cause slowing or stopping of breathing. Your anesthesiologist will take every precaution to minimize the chance that a rare complication will occur.

Pregnant Pause

For some women, although the chance of a serious side effect is very small, the fear of a potential complication is enough to dissuade them from asking for an epidural or spinal. Ultimately, each person must make that decision for herself.

COMPLICATIONS UNRELATED TO REGIONAL PAIN RELIEF

All sorts of troubles are attributed to the epidural or spinal, although in fact they are usually not related. For example, a headache after delivery may have many causes, including lack of sleep or caffeine deprivation. If an epidural or spinal was given, however, all eyes are focused on the anesthesia, and everyone concludes that it must be a post-dural puncture headache (see above).

Similarly, there are many causes of nerve injury during delivery. For example, if the baby's head was pressing on a nerve as it passed through the mother's pelvis during delivery, it could cause postpartum numbness and/or weakness. If forceps were used, they could have irritated a nerve or two. But if the patient received an epidural or spinal, a convenient explanation is simply that the anesthesia must have caused the nerve injury. In fact, although bothersome nerve symptoms may occur after childbirth whether or not an epidural or spinal was used, they nearly always gradually improve with time.

Risks of Not Having Regional Pain Relief

When considering whether to use regional analgesia for childbirth, women and their obstetric caregivers routinely weigh the potential risks of the procedure. This is a sensible approach that should be followed before receiving any treatment or intervention. It is interesting, however, that the risks of *not* receiving regional analgesia are not usually considered. Yet such risks certainly exist.

RISKS OF SYSTEMIC NARCOTIC ANALGESICS

If you choose not to use an epidural or a spinal, and if you are like most women, you will want something to help alleviate the pain of childbirth. Assuming that a "natural" approach doesn't relieve the pain, you are likely to receive a systemic narcotic such as Demerol or morphine. The side effects of such medications—drowsiness, nausea, vomiting and itching—although unpleasant and annoying, are not necessarily risky for the mother. But they may be detrimental to the baby's well-being. For example, narcotics administered to the mother may affect the baby's heart rate, making it difficult to interpret. Systemic narcotics may also cause problems after delivery by slowing down the breathing rate in the newborn. In addition, when compared to babies of mothers who receive epidurals, newborns of mothers who have received systemic narcotics have lower APGAR scores at one minute after birth. APGAR scores are a general measure of neonatal well-being; the higher the score, the better. Babies of mothers who have received systemic narcotics also have a greater likelihood of requiring medication (Narcan) to reverse the effects of the narcotics.

HARMFUL EFFECTS OF UNRELIEVED PAIN
AND THEIR PREVENTION WITH EPIDURALS

In addition to causing suffering, unrelieved pain has many potential harmful consequences for the mother and baby. For example, most mothers hyperventilate during painful contractions, especially if labor breathing techniques are used improperly. Hyperventilation can actually stop the normal drive to breathe between contractions, which can reduce the amount of oxygen in the blood. The mother may develop tingly hands, lightheadedness or even unconsciousness. The baby may be affected as well, since a low level of oxygen in the mother's blood means that less oxygen is transferred through the placenta to the baby. When pain relief is provided by an epidural or spinal, these harmful effects do not occur, and mothers can breathe easily throughout labor and delivery.

Pregnant Pause

Although most pregnant women are aware of at least some of the risks of getting an epidural or a spinal, few mothers-to-be ever consider the risks of *not* getting an epidural or spinal.

There is another reason why the amount of oxygen reaching the baby may be reduced if the mother experiences unrelieved pain. Stressful situations such as severe labor pain cause the body to release adrenaline into the bloodstream. Adrenaline causes narrowing of blood vessels throughout the body, including the blood vessels of the uterus that bring oxygen to the placenta. Therefore, when the mother experiences pain and stress the baby receives less oxygen. Epidurals and spinals stop the pain and thus reduce the adrenaline level in the blood, so the mother's blood vessels do not narrow, allowing more blood (and therefore oxygen) to flow to the placenta and baby. Although for most labors this does not make a difference, it's better for the baby to receive more than less oxygen. Labor is a stressful enough time for the baby as it is.

Another advantage of regional pain relief techniques is that they enable the mother to be in control during the delivery. If you are in excruciating pain, it is much more difficult to comply with the instructions of your obstetrician or midwife. On the other hand, if you are comfortable, you can participate fully and assist your obstetrician or midwife to perform a controlled delivery. This in turn may reduce the trauma to your perineum. A controlled delivery may also be better for your baby. This is especially true for premature babies, who are relatively more fragile than full-term babies: they are likely to be better off if they are delivered in a controlled manner, than if they are forcefully and rapidly expelled from the birth canal.

In addition to decreasing the amount of oxygen transferred from the mother to the baby, unrelieved pain during childbirth may have profoundly unhealthy psychological consequences for the mother. It is becoming increasingly apparent that unrelieved pain and a stressful childbirth may contribute to the development of postpartum psychological trauma. For example, the chance of getting postpartum depression is significantly higher in women who have not received pain relief during childbirth.[9] So effective pain relief, apart from its obvious benefits to alleviate the suffering of labor pain, may also prevent the development of long-lasting psychological trauma.

EPIDURAL USE MAY AVOID GENERAL ANESTHESIA

Another risk of not using an epidural is that you are more likely to require general anesthesia if an unanticipated situation develops during labor that requires an emergency cesarean. If you have an epidural catheter in place, you can usually avoid the need for general anesthesia. Your anesthesiologist can simply administer a stronger dose of local anesthetic through the epidural catheter to numb you completely. By using regional anesthesia, you and your baby avoid the risks of general anesthesia such as failed intubation or aspiration (see Chapter Seven).

It's especially important to have an epidural catheter in place in situations that are known to be associated with a greater chance of needing a forceps or cesarean delivery. For example, for women who are planning a vaginal delivery of twins, or who are attempting to deliver vaginally after a previous cesarean, I strongly recommend the placement of an epidural catheter early during the course of labor.

Pregnant Pause

The psychological effects of unrelieved pain, which have only recently been recognized, should not be underestimated. Unrelieved pain may contribute to the development of postpartum depression, which can have harmful consequences for the new mother and for family dynamics.

Key Concepts to Carry Away

Each woman must weigh the potential benefits of regional pain relief against the potential risks. It is important to keep in mind that apart from ending suffering — certainly reason enough — treating labor pain has other benefits. It reverses the mother's stress response that decreases the supply of blood — and, therefore, oxygen — to the baby. Moreover, there is evidence that pain relief may reduce the chance that the mother will develop postpartum psychological problems. All these reasons are further arguments in favor of selecting an epidural and/or a spinal, the most effective means available to relieve the pain of childbirth.

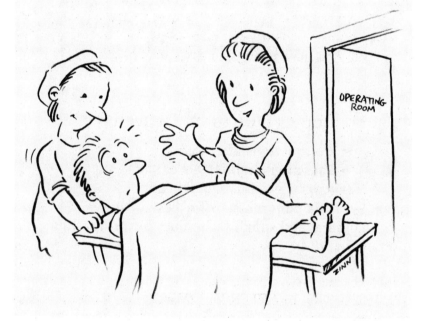

"Mr. Smith, I'll have your hemorrhoid out in 10 minutes. Were you thinking about getting anesthesia today, or did you want to do it naturally?"

9

IT AIN'T OVER TILL IT'S OVER: POSTPARTUM PAIN RELIEF

Topics Due to be Delivered

- **Contractions after delivery**
- **Pain after vaginal delivery**
- **Pain after cesarean delivery**
- **Systemic pain relievers for postpartum pain**
- **Epidural and spinal techniques for postpartum pain**

CONTRACTIONS AFTER DELIVERY

Unfortunately, the pain of childbirth does not end the moment your baby is born, but continues during the postpartum period. Postpartum contractions of the uterus, known as after-pains, occur following both vaginal and cesarean delivery—so don't be surprised when you feel some cramping pain after your baby is born. Following vaginal delivery, women may feel pain in the vaginal and/or perineal area; those who have had cesareans feel other types of pain, mainly from the surgical wound.

AFTER-PAINS

Immediately after the baby and placenta are delivered, the uterus contracts vigorously as it begins the process of shrinking back to its pre-pregnancy size. These postpartum contractions are very important because as the uterus gets smaller, it helps to stop the bleeding from the area where the placenta was attached. The cramping pains of these uterine contractions can be very severe, and tend to get worse with each successive delivery. In fact, some women who have had many babies have told me that their after-pains are even worse than their labor pain.

Pregnant Pause
Although often not taken very seriously by health care providers, after-pains can be quite severe. For some mothers, the after-pains are even worse than the pain of labor itself.

To make matters worse still, Pitocin, a medication that is routinely given as soon as the placenta is delivered to help the uterus to contract, further intensifies the after-pains. Pitocin is administered for a few hours after delivery to minimize blood loss. During breastfeeding, oxytocin, which is the body's natural form of Pitocin, is released from the mother's pituitary gland, causing the after-pains to become very strong. One patient who had three previous deliveries told me that she did not intend to breastfeed her fourth child because she remembered how nursing caused such awful after-pains with her previous baby. I explained that fear of after-pains should not be the reason to avoid breastfeeding, as the pain could be treated using oral medications or by continuing her epidural after delivery (see PCEA after Vaginal Delivery below).

PAIN AFTER VAGINAL DELIVERY

The pain after vaginal delivery varies considerably from one woman to another. Those who have had an easy delivery may only experience mild soreness, while others who have experienced a difficult delivery may have more severe pain. Postpartum pain tends to be worse if forceps were used, if an episiotomy was done or if the tissues of the vagina, perineum and/or anus/rectum were torn.

Evidence now shows that an episiotomy, a controlled surgical incision of the perineum that was often done in order to limit tissue injury during delivery, is usually unnecessary. As a result, fewer obstetricians routinely perform episiotomies anymore, except in specific situations. Regardless of whether or not you have an episiotomy, if the tissues of your perineum are injured, you will have postpartum pain. You may also experience other types of pain after vaginal delivery. For example, hemorrhoids, which are a common occurrence during pregnancy, are often worsened by childbirth.

PAIN AFTER CESAREAN

If you have a cesarean, the postoperative pain can be severe. In addition to cramping pain from uterine contractions (see After-Pains above), you will feel discomfort from the incision itself. This is usually described as a sharp or burning feeling, in comparison to the duller ache of the after-pains. Some women also notice that their shoulders hurt, a condition caused by irritation of the lining of the upper abdomen by blood, amniotic fluid and air within the abdominal cavity.

IMPORTANCE OF POSTPARTUM PAIN RELIEF

Just as there are many advantages to relieving labor pain (see Chapter Eight), it also is important to relieve postpartum pain, to avoid its harmful effects on the mother and newborn. If you are in pain, you will not be able to interact with your newborn as well as you would like to. Unrelieved pain can also lead to medical complications. For example, if pain after a cesarean prevents you from moving around and getting out of bed, you are more likely to develop pneumonia from not breathing deeply, and to develop blood clots from poor circulation. So, in addition to avoiding unnecessary suffering, there are good medical reasons for you to relieve your postpartum pain. Unfortunately, many new mothers mistakenly believe that it is better to avoid pain medication for fear of its effects on the newborn.

EFFECTS OF PAIN MEDICATION ON THE BABY— SYSTEMIC VERSUS REGIONAL APPROACH

If you are nursing, any systemic (i.v. or oral) medication that you take may affect your newborn, as some of it gets passed through your breast milk to the baby. Although this is a relatively tiny percentage of the dose you receive, a newborn can be affected because he or she is so small. If you become drowsy from taking narcotic pain relievers, your breastfeeding baby is likely to be sleepy as well.

Pregnant Pause

Many nursing mothers try to avoid taking pain medication after delivery for fear that it will harm their newborn. If this concerns you, ask to have the epidural continued after delivery — it will keep you comfortable and since the dose is so small, only a tiny amount of medication will be transferred to your baby.

A good way to avoid this is by using regional methods of postpartum pain control. The regional approach makes as much sense for severe postpartum pain as it does for labor pain. Because a smaller dose of medication is given with regional techniques, less is passed to the newborn through your breast milk. If your postpartum pain is relatively mild, you may get by with small doses of systemic pain relievers, for example, Tylenol.

SYSTEMIC NARCOTICS

For many years, the standard method of treating postoperative pain was to inject narcotics like morphine or Demerol into a thigh or arm muscle every few hours. Eventually, the inefficiency of this technique was recognized, as there was too long a delay between the time a patient requested pain medication and the time the drug began to take effect. Intravenous patient-controlled analgesia (PCA) was introduced to avoid this delay.

INTRAVENOUS PATIENT-CONTROLLED ANALGESIA (PCA)

With intravenous PCA, you push a button connected to an electronic pump that triggers a narcotic injection directly into your vein. This eliminates both the time that was once required to call the nurse and have her bring the medication, and the time needed for the medication to travel from the muscle to the brain. Because the narcotic is injected directly into your bloodstream, it reaches your brain very rapidly. The pump, which is the same type used for patient controlled epidural analgesia (PCEA) described in Chapter Five, is programmed so that you cannot overdose yourself. For example, if the pump is programmed for a maximum of one dose every 10 minutes, it will not give you more than that, even if you push the button every minute. There is another safety mechanism that is built-in to PCA techniques. If the narcotic makes you too drowsy to push the button, you will not be able to give yourself any more doses.

Pregnant Pause

Patient-controlled analgesia (PCA) frees the patient from dependence on nurses, who are frequently busy caring for other patients at the same time. An additional benefit is that the freedom to manage one's own pain is empowering.

In many hospitals, pain after cesarean is routinely treated with i.v. PCA narcotics. Although it's clearly better to give narcotics by i.v. PCA than by the old-fashioned way of having a nurse inject the narcotics into a muscle, the disadvantages of systemic narcotics remain: relatively poor pain relief and a high likelihood of side effects.

EPIDURAL AND SPINAL NARCOTICS AFTER CESAREAN

Some hospitals use a regional approach to provide pain relief after a cesarean. In these hospitals, the most common practice is to give a narcotic such as morphine (Duramorph) into the epidural or spinal space. Other drugs have also been used, but morphine has the advantage of being the longest-lasting. A small dose of epidural or spinal morphine given at the time of a cesarean can provide pain relief for as long as 24 hours.

There are some drawbacks to epidural or spinal morphine. For many women, this medication causes side effects including itching, nausea, vomiting, drowsiness and potentially, slow breathing. Other narcotics such as fentanyl and sufentanil are less likely to have these effects, but the pain relief after fentanyl and sufentanil does not last for very long – only two to three hours. Therefore these narcotics are best given repeatedly though an epidural catheter, using patient-controlled epidural analgesia (PCEA; see below).

Pregnant Pause

The most common side effect of epidural or spinal morphine is itching. If this happens to you, your anesthesiologist can treat it with a medication such as Narcan. Giving small doses of Narcan will reverse the narcotic side effects but only minimally affects the pain relief the narcotics provide.

PATIENT-CONTROLLED EPIDURAL ANALGESIA (PCEA) AFTER CESAREAN

An excellent technique of providing pain relief after cesarean is patient-controlled epidural analgesia (PCEA). The epidural catheter is left in place after the operation, delivering a continuous dosage of pain relievers and enabling the mother to self-administer a "booster dose" by pushing a button. The most severe pain following a cesarean occurs on the first day or two, so it's a good idea to use PCEA for approximately 48 hours.

An ideal pain relieving mixture to use for PCEA after cesarean contains a small dose of a local anesthetic combined with a small dose of narcotic. This combination provides excellent pain relief without compromising muscle strength, which is the same principle used for the walking epidural (see Chapter Four). Unlike women who have the walking epidural during labor but usually prefer to rest in bed, women who have had a cesarean are encouraged to get out of bed and walk around. This is not a problem. The pump is attached to the pole on which the intravenous fluid bag is hung. Because the pole is mounted on wheels, the mother can bring her epidural pump with her as she walks (see Figure 3-5). PCEA combines the advantages of excellent pain relief, minimal side effects, and awake and alert mothers who can control their own dosing.

Epidural Episodes:

WHAT A RELIEF

K.V. was a first-time mother who elected to have epidural pain relief. She delivered a beautiful baby boy, but it was as large as it was beautiful — weighing in at 8 pounds 14 ounces. K.V. was 5'2" and had a petite build. So it was not surprising that she ended up with large tear of her perineum. The tear was expertly repaired by her obstetrician immediately after the delivery. Knowing that such an injury hurts considerably, I proposed that K.V. leave the epidural catheter in place and use PCEA for pain control. She was very pleased with the epidural pain relief she had during labor, and readily agreed to the suggestion. For two days after delivery, she received PCEA. It worked well, preventing pain while not making her sleepy. We stopped the PCEA and removed the epidural catheter a few hours before she was scheduled to go home. She noticed the difference within a couple of hours after the flow of medication was stopped. But thanks to the PCEA, she never experienced the worst of the pain that was present for the first 48 hours after delivery.

PATIENT-CONTROLLED EPIDURAL ANALGESIA (PCEA) AFTER VAGINAL DELIVERY

Severe after-pains from uterine contractions and/or significant injury to perineal tissues may cause pain that cannot be adequately treated with oral pain relievers. In these situations I recommend leaving the epidural catheter in place for a day or two to provide pain relief with PCEA. The contraction pains during labor are best relieved by epidurals — so why not relieve postpartum contraction pains the same way? Injury to the tissue of the vagina and perineum can be very painful, so why not use the best type of pain relief available?

Although PCEA provides excellent postpartum pain relief, every technique has its drawbacks. After delivery, some women are bothered by having the catheter in their back and being hooked up to an epidural pump. At some institutions, hospital policy may not allow them to shower if an epidural catheter is in place. I have found that the overwhelming majority of women that I have cared for are so pleased with the quality of pain relief they have received from PCEA, that they willingly put up with the inconvenience of having the catheter in their back.

10

CHILDBIRTH PAIN RELIEF: MYTHS AND REALITIES

Topics Due to be Delivered

- Do epidurals prolong labor?
- Will an epidural interfere with pushing?
- Do epidurals make it more likely that I will need a cesarean?
- Do epidurals make forceps delivery more likely?
- If I move during the epidural placement will I become paralyzed?
- Will the epidural cause a long-lasting backache?
- If I get an epidural, will my baby be affected?
- Will the epidural interfere with breastfeeding?
- Is it ever too early or too late to get an epidural?
- Can I get an epidural if I'm allergic to local anesthetics?
- If I have a slipped disc or if I have had back surgery can I get an epidural?
- Will getting an epidural prevent me from eating or drinking during labor?
- Will the epidural cause a fever that may harm me and my baby?

There are many myths regarding childbirth, and more than a few of these are related to pain relief techniques. Say something often enough, and people will begin to believe it. The way to eradicate such untruths is through education. This chapter reviews commonly held misconceptions about epidurals and spinals with the facts necessary to put them into perspective.

MYTH: "IF I GET AN EPIDURAL, IT WILL SLOW DOWN MY LABOR."

Reality: This is one of the most widely believed epidural myths—nearly everyone I have cared for has been convinced it was true. Women who waited hours before asking for an epidural to relieve their pain often explain that the reason they waited so long was to avoid slowing down their labor. This has been a controversial issue among professionals who care for women during childbirth. Yet, modern regional pain relief actually has little effect on labor's progress. Unfortunately, those who think that it may slow down labor sometimes use it as a pretext to delay or deny epidurals to laboring women.

In 2003, Halpern and Leighton published a review of fourteen studies of the effect of epidurals on labor and delivery that were done between 1980 and 2001.[10] They found that epidurals did not significantly prolong the first stage of labor, and prolonged the second stage of labor by only 15 minutes. An important point to keep in mind is that the epidurals in the studies reviewed used higher doses of local anesthetics—as much as five times higher—than the local anesthetic doses used for today's walking epidural. It stands to reason that the higher the local anesthetic dose, the more muscle weakness will be produced, and the more likely that the second (pushing) stage will be prolonged. Yet even if we take the results of Halpern and Leighton's analysis at face value, should a 15 minute prolongation of labor dissuade you from receiving the most effective method of pain relief for childbirth? Interestingly, obstetricians and patients have told me that on many occasions the administration of the epidural sped up labor. I am no more convinced of that than of the claim that epidurals slow the process, leading us to a basic truth: Labor can never pass quickly enough, but an epidural always makes it less painful.

MYTH: "IF I HAVE AN EPIDURAL, I WON'T BE ABLE TO PUSH WELL."

Reality: During the first stage of labor, the uterine contractions dilate the cervix. During the second stage of labor, you have a much more active role — you help to push the baby out. As mentioned above, the second stage of labor may be prolonged on average by about 15 minutes in women who get epidurals, suggesting that the epidural somehow hinders pushing. Keep in mind that this conclusion was based on studies that used much higher doses of local anesthetic than are used in today's walking epidurals — so it all depends on the type of epidural that you have.

There are two ways that an epidural could prevent you from pushing effectively — by blocking the pressure sensation as the baby descends and/or by causing muscle weakness.

An epidural that is working very well may completely block the feeling of pressure that normally occurs as the baby descends towards the birth canal. Most women, especially those delivering their first baby, find that it is easier to push effectively when they are able to feel this pressure — it serves as a focus for their pushing efforts. If the epidural eliminates this pressure sensation entirely, it may be more difficult for you to push effectively. This often occurred with the old-fashioned high-dose epidurals. Ideally, the epidural will relieve your pain but leave you with a feeling of pressure during the second stage. If the epidural causes your muscles to be weak, it may be more difficult for you to push the baby out, thereby prolonging the second stage.

The walking epidural aims to minimize muscle weakness while

preserving the sensation of pressure. It does this by using very
low doses of local anesthetics. Also, because the walking
epidural affects pain nerves more than it affects the nerves that
control muscle function, you retain the strength needed to push
effectively. With patient-controlled epidural analgesia (PCEA),
the mother-to-be can fine-tune the amount of pain relievers she
receives, so that she can adjust the intensity of her pain relief to
the point where the pain is blocked but muscle strength and the
pressure sensation are maintained.

MYTH: "IF I GET AN EPIDURAL, I AM MORE LIKELY TO NEED A CESAREAN."

Reality: The myth that epidurals lead to an increased likelihood
of cesarean still exists despite considerable evidence to the contrary. Although numbers alone may indicate that there is an
association between epidurals and cesarean delivery, closer
examination of the data show that epidurals do not cause
cesareans. Think about it—women who have difficult, prolonged labors and end up having a cesarean also tend to have
more painful labors (see Chapter Five). Thus, these women are

more likely to request and receive epidurals—but their epidurals did not cause their cesareans. They would have needed a cesarean in any event. So one cannot simply compare epidural rates and cesarean rates and conclude that epidurals caused the cesareans.

In a 1997 New York Times article on the subject, an obstetrician, Dr. John Thorp, summarized the roots of this myth well: "There's a problem with the way the literature has been interpreted. There is a strong association between epidurals and Cesareans, but not causality. Epidurals that were placed after an abnormal labor occurred can't be blamed for Cesareans."[11] Yet despite the evidence, the myth persists.

MYTH: "IF I GET AN EPIDURAL, I'M MORE LIKELY TO NEED A FORCEPS DELIVERY."

Reality: Forceps deliveries tend to occur more frequently in patients who receive epidurals, but do epidurals cause forceps deliveries? Like cesarean deliveries (see previous myth) it is not surprising that there is an association between epidurals and forceps deliveries. But it is not at all clear that using an epidural adversely affects labor so that forceps become necessary. Women with dysfunctional labors—labors that are destined not to progress well, for whatever reason, are more likely to experience pain (see Chapter Five). Therefore, these women are more likely to request an epidural. That these same women end up with a higher rate of forceps delivery is no surprise. In other words, the women who have more intense labor pain are likely to have a smaller chance of experiencing an easy vaginal delivery regardless of whether or not they received an epidural. The epidural is given to relieve the pain, and then it is blamed for the use of forceps that would probably have been needed anyway.

If the epidural prevents effective pushing (see above), it stands to reason that epidurals would increase the rate of forceps delivery. Because the low-dose walking epidural tends to preserve the ability to push, it should be associated with lower rates of forceps deliveries. There is now some evidence for this. A study of 1,054 patients showed that low-dose epidural techniques resulted in a lower likelihood of the need for forceps deliveries than did traditional higher-dose epidurals. In fact, the authors concluded, "...continued routine use of traditional epidurals might not be justified."[12] Clearly, low-dose walking epidurals make sense. And using PCEA (see above) makes even more sense.

MYTH: "IF I MOVE WHEN THE EPIDURAL NEEDLE IS BEING PLACED, I CAN BE PARALYZED."

Reality: This is one of the most commonly expressed fears of patients who are contemplating an epidural. It's difficult to remain completely still while you are feeling an excruciating contraction pain. In fact, you are expected to move during severe labor pain; most of my patients are moving around quite a bit when I insert their epidural. Despite this, I have never seen a labor epidural cause paralysis. In reality, if you were to suddenly move during the procedure, the worst result would likely be a spinal headache if the needle were to make a hole in the dura (see Chapter Eight). Unfortunately, many patients believe that this myth is true, and it causes a lot of unnecessary worry.

MYTH: "IF I HAVE AN EPIDURAL, I WILL END UP WITH A BACKACHE."

Reality: For many women, the prospect of backache during pregnancy and after delivery is worrisome. Backache is common during pregnancy, as a result of the stress the weight of the baby puts on the muscles and ligaments of the spine. Some women who are fortunate to get through pregnancy without backache may develop it during labor and delivery. Thus, many mothers end up with a backache after delivery that may last for a long time – weeks to months. Not surprisingly, if they had an epidural, they may blame the pain relief technique for their backache—"I was fine before I had that needle in my back." However, careful scientific investigation of this issue has clearly shown that epidurals do not cause backaches. The chance of developing a long-lasting backache is identical whether or not an epidural is used.

MYTH: "IF I GET AN EPIDURAL, IT WILL INTERFERE WITH BREASTFEEDING."

Reality: It's never been proven that epidurals interfere with breastfeeding, although some proponents of breastfeeding argue this point passionately. It is true that any medication that you take to relieve your pain will in fact reach the baby—including medication administered though your epidural or spinal. However, with an epidural the amount of drug that enters your bloodstream is quite small. With a spinal, the amount is even smaller. One of the components used in walking epidural techniques is a very low dose of synthetic narcotic. Some have voiced concern that the narcotic will have an adverse effect on the newborn, and will compromise its ability to breast-feed. But scientific evidence does not support this view. Insofar as we can tell, there is no effect of modern low-dose walking epidurals on the newborn's ability to breastfeed, but better-designed studies of this issue are needed. Contrast this with the effects that systemic pain relievers taken by the mother may have on the baby. Morphine or Demerol makes the mother sleepy, and the breastfeeding baby becomes sleepy as well.

MYTH: IF IT IS "TOO EARLY" OR "TOO LATE," YOU CAN'T GET AN EPIDURAL.

Reality: A very common misconception is that epidurals can only be given when the cervix is dilated to a certain number of centimeters. However, this concept of a "window of opportunity" for receiving pain relief during labor has no validity. In fact, an epidural may be administered at any time once labor has been diagnosed or a decision to deliver the baby has been made—even before the cervix begins to dilate—to the end of labor, when the cervix is completely dilated. This issue and controversies surrounding the timing of epidural and spinal pain relief are discussed fully in Chapter Five.

MYTH: NO PAIN, NO GAIN.

Reality: While this may or may not be true for an exercise program, this notion is patently false for labor. Can you imagine this argument being made to a man about to undergo "minor" surgery for hemorrhoids? In a 1999 New York Times Magazine article, Margaret Talbot, who underwent both a "natural" and an epidural labor experience, wrote that "Today's natural-childbirth purists...regard labor as an extreme sport—an ennobling physical challenge that we pampered First Worlders are supposed to courageously endure and savor. Spurning the palliatives of modern medicine is part of the drill, an emblem of virtue....Yet what matters, surely, is not how you get through labor but that you get through it." [13]

MYTH: "I HAVE AN ALLERGY TO LOCAL ANES- THETICS SO I CAN'T GET AN EPIDURAL."

Reality: True allergy to a local anesthetic is rare. Most of the time, women relate a story in which they have had some type of bad reaction to a local anesthetic at the dentist's office. In many cases, the perceived "allergy" may be explained by a small amount of adrenaline, which is often added to the local anesthetic, being injected into a blood vessel. This typically causes very unpleasant symptoms including trembling and a feeling that your heart is racing. But it is unlikely that this reaction was caused by a true allergy to the local anesthetic.

The other main component of regional pain relief is a synthetic narcotic. Allergies to synthetic narcotics are also rare, so it is highly unlikely that you would be allergic to this type of medication. It is possible for you to be tested before you go into labor to see if you have true allergies to any of the pain relievers that you may receive, although the tests themselves are not 100% accurate. If you are concerned about a potential allergy to a pain reliever, you should discuss it with an anesthesiologist long in advance of your due date, so that a consultation with an allergist can be obtained, and a plan can be devised.

MYTH: "I CAN'T HAVE AN EPIDURAL BECAUSE I HAVE A HERNIATED DISC."

Reality: Having a herniated or bulging disc does not mean that you can't get an epidural. In fact, many people with herniated discs are actually treated with epidural injections. A common misconception is that if there is already a problem in the lower back, why chance worsening it by putting a needle there? In fact, the discs that are located between the vertebrae of the spine are located on the front side of the dura. Because an epidural is performed from behind the spine, the needle does not even get near the disc (see Figures 3-1 and 3-2). One reason that some anesthesiologists avoid using an epidural in a woman with a disc problem is the fear that the epidural will be wrongly blamed if the symptoms happen to worsen afterward. The fact is that delivery itself may worsen the symptoms of a herniated or bulging disc whether or not an epidural is used. So the good news is that if you have a disc problem and you want an epidural, it's no problem. Other back problems such as scoliosis should not prevent you from getting an epidural either. In fact, many women who have undergone major back surgery have received epidurals for labor pain relief.

MYTH: "I CAN'T EAT OR DRINK ONCE I HAVE THE EPIDURAL."

Reality: Having the epidural does not limit your right to eat or drink, but being in labor does. This is for safety's sake because the course and outcome of labor are not predictable, and there is a chance that you may require general anesthesia for an emergency cesarean. Thus, it is best that your stomach be relatively empty because aspiration—the spilling of stomach contents into the lungs (see Chapter Seven)—is a serious event. Aspiration of solid food substances is more damaging than aspiration of liquids. So once you're in labor, you shouldn't have solid foods at all. The old-fashioned approach was to avoid liquids as well, but the thinking on this one has changed. It's certainly much more pleasant if you can have something to drink if you're thirsty. Nowadays, it's generally acceptable that a woman in labor be allowed to drink moderate amounts of clear liquids, that is, liquids that don't contain solid particles— whether or not she has an epidural.

MYTH: "EPIDURALS CAUSE FEVERS THAT WILL HARM ME AND MY BABY."

Reality: Since 1987, an association between the use of epidural pain relief and a rise in the mother's temperature has been recognized. Although the cause of the temperature rise is not entirely clear, it appears to be related to the amount of time the epidural is in place. There doesn't seem to be any effect for the first four to five hours of epidural use, but afterward the mother's temperature increases approximately 0.2° Fahrenheit per hour. While it is unlikely that an increased temperature in the mother is dangerous, it may be misinterpreted as a sign of infection and lead to tests being done on the mother and newborn to determine if an infection is truly present. It may even prompt physicians to administer antibiotics to the mother and newborn. These are the concerns — that the baby will have to undergo tests or receive unnecessary antibiotics.

If the mother's temperature does rise, it presents a challenge to physicians caring for her and her baby. This is where clinical judgment is important, and the decision to perform diagnostic tests and to give antibiotics must be based on the entire clinical picture — not only on the mother's temperature. There are many harmless causes of a raised temperature, for example, exercising. Just because the mother received an epidural doesn't mean that diagnostic tests must be done on her newborn.

Key Concepts to Carry Away

There are many misconceptions about epidural and spinal pain relief. Be sure that you know the difference between myth and reality. Being knowledgeable will help you to decide on the type of pain relief (if any) you will want. Also, knowing the facts should help to decrease your anxiety about epidurals and spinals.

11

CONTEMPLATING
PAIN-FREE LABOR

Old ideas die hard. Long after forward-thinkers had proved that the earth was round, flat earth societies continued to flourish. In every field of human endeavor, it takes a long time before people feel comfortable with new concepts. Change is difficult to accept. The subject of relief of childbirth pain is no exception. Although more than 150 years have passed since the first anesthetic for childbirth was given, many people continue to believe that women are meant to experience pain during labor and delivery. Although pain-free delivery that is safe for both mother and baby is possible with state-of-the-art epidurals and spinals, many women continue to suffer through the experience, primarily out of fear, guilt and ignorance.

My goal in writing this book has been to make available the facts about modern pain relief for childbirth, and to demystify the techniques in use today, in order to help you decide whether you want to make use of these medical miracles during your delivery. I sincerely hope that, in so doing, I have addressed your fears and concerns. If I have encouraged you to seek further information and to consult with your obstetrician or midwife and anesthesiologist well in advance of your labor, then I have succeeded in my task. Ultimately, it is your right alone to decide the type of pain relief—if any—that you would like to receive. Keep in mind, however, that if you choose an epidural or a spinal, you truly can ENJOY YOUR LABOR!

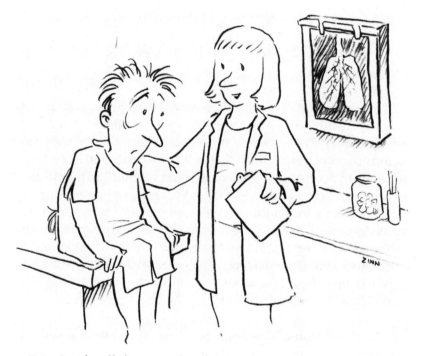

"Mr. Smith, all the tests show that you have pneumonia—so which will it be: penicillin or the natural approach?"

NOTES

1. Berrin K, Seligman TK. *Art of the Huichol Indians.* Harry N. Abrams, Inc. New York. 1978, p. 162.

2. Brownridge P, *European Journal of Obstetrics Gynecology and Reproductive Biology.* 1995 May; 59 Suppl:S9-15.

3. Wagenknecht EC. *Mrs. Longfellow: Selected Letters and Journals of Fanny Appleton Longfellow (1817-1861).* New York: Longmire Green & Co.; 1956:129-130.

4. Caton, D. *What a Blessing She Had Chloroform: The Medical and Social Response to the Pain of Childbirth from 1800 to the Present.* New Haven: Yale University Press, 1999, p.127.

5. Caton, D. *What a Blessing She Had Chloroform: The Medical and Social Response to the Pain of Childbirth from 1800 to the Present.* New Haven: Yale University Press, 1999, p.24.

6. Wong CA, Scavone BM, Peaceman AM, McCarthy RJ, Sullivan JT, Diaz NT, Yaghmour E, Marcus RJ, Sherwani SS, Sproviero MT, Yilmaz M, Patel R, Robles C, Grouper S. The risk of cesarean delivery with neuraxial analgesia given early versus late in labor. *New England Journal of Medicine* 2005; 352:655-665.

7. Wuitchik M, Bakal D, Lipshitz J. The clinical significance of pain and cognitive activity in latent labor. *Obstetrics and Gynecology* 1989; 73:35-42.

8. American College of Obstetricians and Gynecologists. ACOG Committee Opinion: Analgesia and cesarean delivery rates. *International Journal of Gynecology and Obstetrics* 2002; 77:297-298.

9. Hiltunen P, Raudaskoski T, Ebeling H, Moilanen I. Does pain relief during delivery decrease the risk of postnatal depression? *Acta Obstetrica and Gynecologica Scandinavica* 2004; 83:257-261.

10. Halpern SH, Leighton BL. Misconceptions about neuraxial analgesia. *Anesthesiology Clinics of North America*. 2003; 21:59-70.

11. Gilbert, S. No Cesarean Risk Is Found For a Labor Pain Medication. *New York Times*. October 21, 1997, p. F9.

12. Comparative Obstetric Mobile Epidural Trial (COMET). Effect of low-dose mobile versus traditional epidural techniques on mode of delivery: a randomised controlled trial. Study Group UK. *Lancet*. 2001; 358:19-23.

13. Talbot, M. Pay on Delivery. *New York Times Magazine* October 31, 1999, pp. 19-20.

GLOSSARY

ACOG – American College of Obstetricians and Gynecologists. It has over 46,000 members and is the nation's leading group of professionals providing health care for women.

Adrenaline (epinephrine) – A chemical produced in the adrenal glands, especially during times of stress. Among other effects, adrenaline narrows blood vessels, including those of the uterus, thus reducing the amount of oxygen that is brought to the baby.

After-pains – Abdominal pains due to contractions of the uterus after the baby is born, which are worsened by breast-feeding; they tend to increase in severity with each successive birth.

Analgesia – The relief of pain without the loss of consciousness.

Anesthesia – The loss of pain sensation as in surgery, with or without the loss of consciousness.

APGAR – A scoring system to rate the well-being of a baby during the first few minutes of life; devised by American anesthesiologist Virginia Apgar.

Aspiration – The spilling of stomach contents into the lungs as may occur in an unconscious person.

Asphyxia – the condition in which there is a lack of oxygen and a build up of carbon dioxide leading to loss of consciousness or death.

Birth canal – The lower potion of the uterus, the cervix and the vagina through which the baby passes during delivery.

Bonding – The process in which a close, loving relationship develops between the baby and the parents after birth.

Bradycardia – Slow heart rate.

Breech – The baby's position in the uterus where the feet or buttocks are poised to emerge first, before the head.

Cervix – The opening at the outlet of the uterus through which the baby passes during the delivery.

Combined spinal-epidural (CSE) – A regional pain relief technique in which both a spinal and an epidural are performed at the same time.

Dilate, dilation – The widening of a structure to a larger size.

Dura – A layer of tissue that covers the brain and spinal cord, and surrounds the spinal fluid.

EKG (electrocardiogram) – A recording of the electrical activity of the heart; used to monitor heart function.

Electronic infusion pump – A device that can be programmed to give a specific dose of medication. It may be used to provide a steady dose and/or to give intermittent doses in response to patient need. See patient controlled analgesia (PCA) and patient controlled epidural analgesia (PCEA).

Epidural – A space within the vertebral column, outside the dura, through which nerves travel. Also, the anesthetic technique in which medication is injected to block the pain signal from traveling through the nerves, to keep the patient pain-free and awake.

Epidural blood patch – A procedure to treat post-spinal headaches, in which approximately one-half ounce of the patient's blood is taken from a forearm vein, and is injected into the epidural space. The blood forms a clot that seals the hole in the dura, which prevents the further leakage of spinal fluid. See also Spinal headache.

Epidural catheter – A tiny soft, flexible plastic tube through which pain relieving medications are injected into the epidural space.

Epidural needle – A specially designed needle that is placed into the epidural space in order to inject medications and/or fluids, and through which an epidural catheter may be passed.

Epinephrine – See Adrenaline.

Episiotomy – A controlled surgical incision of the perineum performed by the obstetrician to limit the tearing of tissues during the delivery of the baby.

First stage of labor – See stages of labor.

Forceps – Instruments sometimes used by the obstetrician to help deliver the baby.

Hyperventilation – Rapid breathing

Intravenous (i.v.) – Literally "in the vein," it refers to the needle or small plastic tube that is placed into a vein to administer fluids and/or medications.

i.v. – See Intravenous

Intubation – The act of inserting a plastic tube into the trachea (windpipe) in order to administer oxygen and anesthetic gases.

Midazolam (Versed) – A medication related to Valium that may be given through the i.v., which produces sedation and relieves anxiety.

Obstetric anesthesiologist – An anesthesiologist who provides pain relief for labor and delivery, and in the postpartum period.

Occiput posterior – the position in which the baby's head is delivered facing toward the ceiling; may be associated with more painful labor, especially in the lower back.

Oxytocin – See Pitocin.

Patient controlled analgesia (PCA) – A technique in which the patient controls her own dosing of pain relievers that are injected into her i.v. by pushing a button connected to an electronic infusion pump. The pump is programmed to prevent overdosing.

Patient controlled epidural analgesia (PCEA) – A technique in which the patient controls her own dosing of pain relievers that are injected into her epidural catheter by pushing a button connected to an electronic infusion pump. The pump is programmed to prevent overdosing,

Perineum (perineal area) – The region between the vagina and the anus.

Pitocin – A synthetic form of the hormone oxytocin; given by the obstetrician to cause uterine contractions.

Post-dural puncture headache – See spinal headache.

Post partum – The interval after the delivery of the baby.

Pulse oximeter – A small device that is placed on a finger to measure the amount of oxygen in the blood.

Regional pain relief – The technique of administering pain relieving medication to eliminate pain in a specific area (region) of the body; for example, epidurals and spinals.

Resuscitation – Restoring breathing and blood circulation to a patient in distress.

Second stage of labor – See stages of labor.

Spinal – The term used to describe pain relief that is achieved by injecting medication into the cerebrospinal fluid.

Spinal cord – The cluster of nerves located within the vertebral column through which signals are transmitted from the body to the brain.

Spinal fluid – The fluid surrounding and cushioning the brain and spinal cord.

Spinal headache – Also called post-dural puncture headache. It results from the leakage of cerebrospinal fluid through a hole in the dura created by a spinal or epidural needle.

Spinous processes – The parts of the spinal bones that can be felt as a small bumps along the center of the back. The anesthesiologist feels these bumps in order to determine precisely where to place the epidural or spinal needle.

Stages of labor –
   First Stage – The portion of labor from the onset of regular contractions, which cause the cervix to change shape, until full dilation of the cervix (ten centimeters) is reached.
   Second Stage – The portion of labor from full dilation of the cervix until the delivery of the baby.
   Third Stage – The interval from the birth of the baby to the delivery of the placenta.

Stat – Immediately

Synthetic narcotic – A man-made pain reliever similar in chemical structure and function to morphine.

Systemic pain relief – The technique in which pain relieving medication is administered into a vein, a muscle or taken by mouth, and is then distributed throughout the entire body (system).

Trachea (windpipe) – The tubular structure in the neck through which air from the mouth and nose travels to the lungs.

Third stage of labor – See stages of labor.

Uterus – The womb; the pelvic organ in which the baby grows.

Versed – see Midazolam.

Walking epidural – A technique in which a low-dose of a local anesthetic, usually combined with a synthetic narcotic, is given to produce pain relief with a minimum of muscle weakness, to enable the mother to walk if she desires, and to push effectively during the second stage of labor.

INDEX

booster doses, 33. See also PCEA

bradycardia (slowing of baby's heart rate), 68; and cesarean, 55

breast engorgement, 62

breastfeeding: and after-pains, 79-80; and epidural, 91

breathing tube, 54

Brownridge, Dr. Peter, 9

butorphanol. See Stadol

caffeine deprivation, and headache, 71

catheter, urinary 68

Caton, Dr. Donald: *What a Blessing She Had Chloroform: The Medical and Surgical Response to the Pain of Childbirth from 1800 to the Present*, 19

"caudal" procedure, 21-23

cervix: dilation of, 12, 37–38; and dysfunctional labor, 40-41; and timing of epidural, 39, 40, 41, 91

cesarean, 32, 40, 53-60, 66; and anesthesiologist's procedure, 57-59; and blood pressure, 58; and causing of, with epidural, 88; and general anesthesia, 58; and general vs. regional anesthesia, 54–56; and epidural and spinal narcotics after, 81-82; and mobility, 82; and obstetrician's procedure, 58, 59, 60; and PCA, 80-81; and PCEA, 82; and perception of failure, 60; and postoperative pain, 79; and strength of anesthetic dosage with, 56; and timing of epidural, 37-39

cesarean, stat (emergency), 53-54

Channing, Dr. Walter, 19

childbirth education classes, 1

childbirth, natural. See natural childbirth

childbirth pain: and double standard, 5; and Huichol Indians, 6; and prejudice, 6

childbirth pain relief: and chloroform gas, 18; and ether, 18; and feelings of guilt, 9; history of, 17–30; natural or unnatural, 6–8; and opposition to, 18, 19; perceptions of, 5–10; vs. natural childbirth, 19

chloroform, 18, 19

combined spinal-epidural, 27, 28 (figure 3-7), 31, 32, 33, 56-57

complications, local and systemic, 73–74

contractions: after delivery, 77–78, 83; compared to menstrual cramps, 12; and intravenous fluids, 67; and systemic nar-

epidural needle, 21-23, 22 (figure 3-2), 47, 49-51; size of, 63-64 (figure 8-1)

epidural space, 21-23, 24 (figure 3-4), 31, 49

episiotomy, 78-79

ether: in favor of use of, 18; history of, 18–19; objections to, in childbirth, 18, 19

feelings of guilt about pain relief, 8-10

fentanyl, in epidural, 31, 82

fever and epidural, 94

first stage of labor, 11–12. See also labor, stages of

fluids, intravenous. See intravenous fluids

forceps: and dysfunctional labor, 40, 89; and incidence of use with epidural, 40, 41, 89; and progress of labor, 38; and saddle block, 41

"funny-bone" sensation, 50

general anesthesia, 54-56, 58, 59

Genesis 3:16, and objections to pain relief in childbirth, 18-19

guilt feelings. See feelings of guilt about pain relief

headache, 74. See also spinal headache

heart rate of baby: and emergency cesarean, 53

herniated disc, and epidural, 93

higher-dose epidurals, 90

history: of epidurals, 21–25, 29; of ether, 17-18; of pain relief in childbirth, 17–28

Huichol Indians, and birth customs, 6–7

hyperventilation, dangers of, 72-73

inability to urinate, 68

infection. See rare risks of epidurals and spinals

intravenous fluids: and epidurals, 66; and low blood pressure, 67

need to urinate, and intravenous fluids, 67
nerve damage. See rare risks of epidurals and spinals

Stadol (butorphanol), 13, 21
stat (*statim*), 53-54
sufentanil, 31
supine hypotensive syndrome, 67. See also decreased blood
    pressure; regional pain relief, risks of
synthetic narcotics, 31

Thorp, Dr. John, and myth of epidurals causing cesareans, 89
third stage of labor, 12
transition stage (of labor), 12
twilight sleep, 20

urinary catheter, 68
uterine contractions. See contractions
unnatural childbirth. See childbirth, natural

vagina, during labor, 12
vena cava, and low blood pressure, 67
vertebral column, 22 (figure 3-1), 26 (figure 3-5)
Versed (midazolam), 60

walking epidural, 24, 25 (figure 3-5), 29-30, and low dosage, 87;
    muscle weakness, and pressure, 87-88, and newborn's abili-
    ty to breastfeed, 91; and PCEA, 33-35
weakness, postpartum, 71
"window of opportunity," 37
Wong, Dr. Cynthia, 38
Wuitchik, Dr. Michael, 40

ABOUT THE AUTHOR

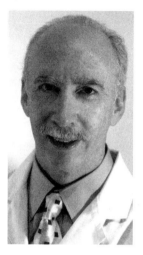

Dr. Gilbert J. Grant earned his MD degree from the University of Michigan Medical School in 1982. He then moved to New York City, where he completed an internship in Obstetrics and Gynecology at Columbia Presbyterian Hospital and a residency in anesthesiology at New York University Medical Center. Dr. Grant then joined the staff of the Department of Anesthesiology of New York University Medical Center where he is currently Associate Professor, Director of Obstetric Anesthesia, and Vice Chairman for Academic Affairs.

In addition to his medical practice, Dr. Grant has continuously been engaged in clinical and laboratory research focused on improving patient care. He was an active participant in the changeover from the "old-fashioned" epidural in vogue at the beginning of his career to the "walking" epidural that he now routinely administers. Since 1989 he has worked on developing an ultra-long-acting local anesthetic designed to provide sustained pain relief. Dr. Grant has published numerous scientific papers and chapters for medical textbooks, and he lectures at educational institutions and scientific meetings in the United States and abroad.

Proprietary pharmaceuticals mentioned in this book:

Trade Name	*Generic Name*	*Manufacturer*
Betadine	providone iodine	Purdue Pharma, L.P.
Demerol	meperidine	Sanofi-Synthelabo, Inc.
Duramorph	preservative-free morphine	Elkins-Sinn, Inc.
Narcan	naloxone	Endo Pharmaceuticals
Nubain	nalbuphine	Endo Pharmaceuticals
Stadol	butorphanol	Geneva Pharmaceuticals, Inc.
Tylenol	acetaminophen	McNeil Consumer & Specialty Pharmaceuticals
Valium	diazepam	Roche Pharmaceuticals
Versed	midazolam	Roche Pharmaceuticals

HELP SOMEONE YOU KNOW
TO ENJOY THEIR LABOR!

Order additional copies of
Enjoy Your Labor: A New Approach to Pain Relief for Childbirth

$14.95 each

Add $3.00 shipping (Ground) and handling for one book,
and $1.00 for each additional book.

My check or money order for $_____ is enclosed.

Name _____

Organization _____

Street Address _____

City/State/Zip _____

Phone _____

Email_____

Make checks payable and return to:
Russell Hastings Press, Ltd.
P.O. Box 229
White Plains, NY 10605

Please allow 2–3 weeks for delivery

For more rapid shipping options, and/or to charge your book
to a major credit card, order online at:
www.EnjoyYourLabor.com

For bulk orders, contact:
sales@RussellHastingsPress.com